P9-CRH-736

TIME OUT!

A PARENTS' GUIDE TO UNDERSTANDING AND DEALING WITH CHALLENGING CHILDREN

MALIN ALFVÉN & KRISTINA HOFSTEN

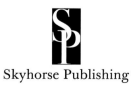

Skyhorse Publishing

copyright © 2015 by malin alfvén and kristina hofsten

all rights reserved. no part of this book may be reproduced in any manner without the express written consent of the publisher, except in the case of brief excerpts in critical reviews or articles. all inquiries should be addressed to skyhorse publishing, 307 west 36th street, 11th floor, new york, ny 10018.

skyhorse publishing books may be purchased in bulk at special discounts for sales promotion, corporate gifts, fund-raising, or educational purposes. special editions can also be created to specifications. for details, contact the special sales department, skyhorse publishing, 307 west 36th street, 11th floor, new york, ny 10018 or info@skyhorsepublishing.com.

skyhorse® and skyhorse publishing® are registered trademarks of skyhorse publishing, inc.®, a delaware corporation.

visit our website at www.skyhorsepublishing.com.

10 9 8 7 6 5 4 3 2 1

library of congress cataloging-in-publication data is available on file.

print isbn: 978-1-62914-729-1
ebook isbn: 978-1-62914-881-6

printed in china

Time Out!

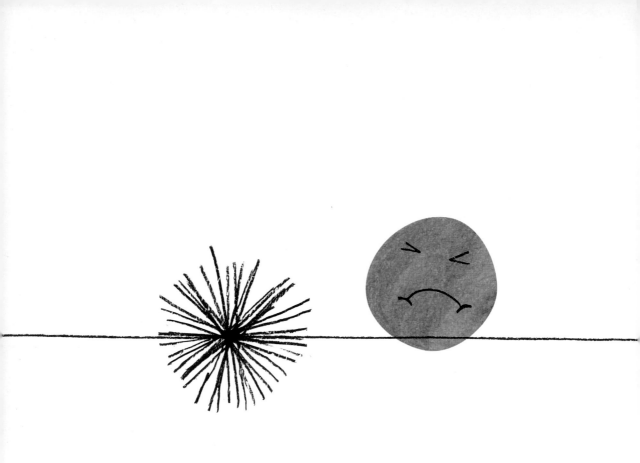

Contents

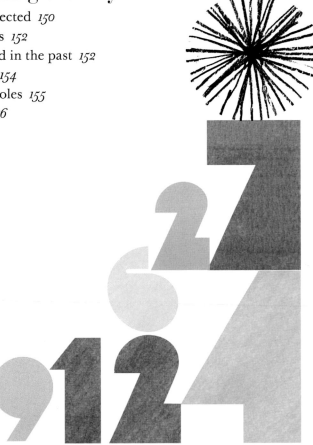

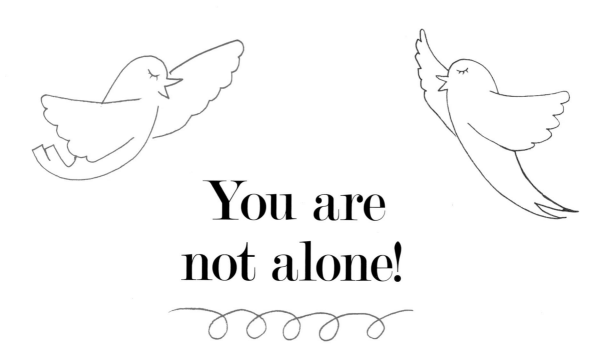

You are not alone!

When you are in the middle of a "parent-child crisis," it is nice to get hands-on advice and feel that you are not alone. And it is nice to laugh a little.

Thanks to child psychiatrist Göran Höberg, social worker Eva Gunnarskog, and pediatrician Gösta Alfvén, who helped us with their experiences with children and adolescents.

And thank you to all parents and children who came forward with their situations and shared their thoughts and emotions.

Malin Alfvén and Kristina Hofsten

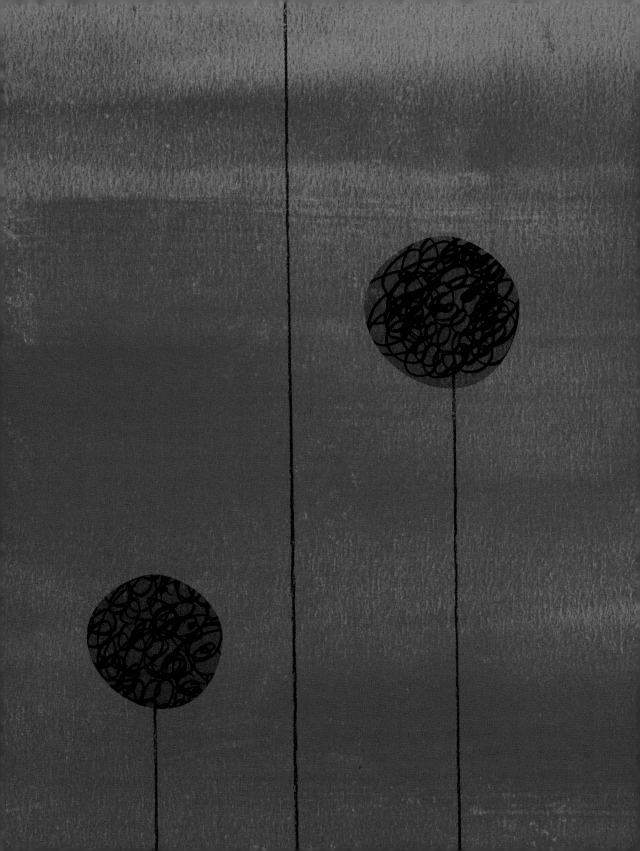

Defiance
and maturity

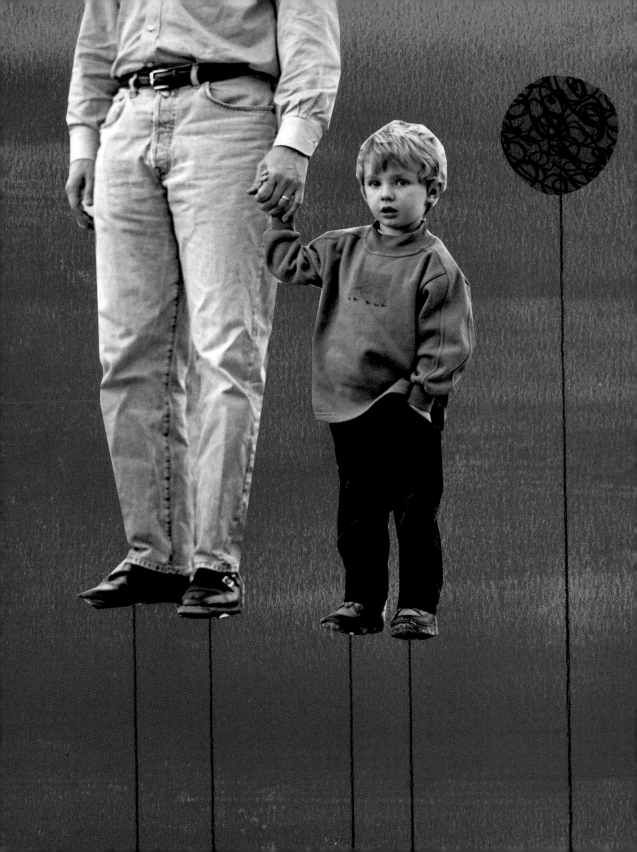

"HE HAS ENTERED THE DEFIANCE AGE," parents sigh when the child suddenly becomes frustrated, awkward, defiant, or angry, and generally impossible. As if there was only one single defiance age! In fact, life is composed of many different periods of defiance. And this is how it should be, because defiance leads to maturity and development. We might even say that defiance and development go hand in hand, that both are needed. Just like a little four-year-old girl who fought a lot with her mom said: "I feel in my heart that I need to fight with you." So there is nothing wrong when the child suddenly becomes defiant. But nevertheless, it can be very difficult. We do not know how we should act towards our children. What used to work so well in the past, now does not work at all. We do not recognize our child. We worry about how our difficult child will get along with other children and adults, how she will be treated. We feel we've failed.

Defiance is something we do throughout life

Throughout life, we all enter into more or less intensive periods of maturity when we become defiant and say "No, I will not." Though, we

13

say it in different ways at different ages. Already during our first year, we go through at least seven phases of development. We all know about the two and three-year-olds' defiance age. New phases of defiance and development occur at about four, six, nine, and twelve years of age, and of course, in adolescence. This continues throughout life. Pregnancy is such a time of development, crisis, and maturity, mostly for the woman but also for the man who is about to become a father.

And what are the thirty-year and forty-year crises if not important stages of development? For women, menopause is a crisis and a period of transition. Retirement is a tumultuous time for all of us, just like the idea of "moving to the assisted home." In short, we defy and develop throughout life. Children are very different from each other; they differ just as adults do in temperament and way of being. To speak of a typical two-year-old or six-year-old is just as mad as to speak of a typical thirty-two-year-old or forty-eight-year-old. We are individuals and want to be treated as such. Individuality cannot be tucked away in age bins.

Nevertheless, we broadly follow the same physical development. We learn to crawl and stand, walk and talk, all in this order and at about the same age. Some years later, we are mature enough to learn how to ride a bike and skate. Similarly, we all go through a spiritual development. It is not always quiet and smooth but more typically it happens in sudden leaps, and we oscillate between calmer and more troubled periods. How vigorously and how often we oscillate depends partly on heredity, environment, and external events. For children these periods occur at about the same age, although it somewhat varies depending on how early or late the child is in his development as a whole. Some children start their two-year-old's crisis before the age of two, other children start at three. The six-year-old's perhaps occurs half a year before or six months after the child turns six.

A starting point for something new

All these periods of defiance and maturity mean both a summation and a starting point for something new. We grow and change our ways.

We defy both ourselves and our environment. We often become more sensitive and cry easily. There is a reason to it. We need to take care of the feelings we have, both the positive and the negative.

Each defiance age is about opposites. We are happy and sad, gentle and angry, awkward and cuddly. We want to be both independent and dependent. We could say: we are everything we usually are and can be, but with much more intensity than usual. For many, defiance can have a negative connotation. Nevertheless, defiance is something necessary and good. It leads to something positive. Each defiance age opens up the world more and more. Instead of defiance age, we could call it developmental age or maturity period, or "I-want-to-and-can-do-it-myself-period."

When the intensive developmental phase has toned down, a calmer period of recovery follows. It is usually called the harmonious five and ten years of age. It is as if one gets back the child one had before the defiance age, though more mature. The stormy time is over and it is a relief. We can finally harvest the fruits, until the child falls into a new defiance age.

How severely the child reacts varies. Some children enter each defiance age with full force, while in others you hardly notice the periods of crisis. One never knows. Suddenly, the calm and "nice" child who never reacted at nine months or even two or four years, enters a hefty six-year-old's crisis.

Sensitive children (and adults) react more than others when they enter the defiance ages. They have a strong responsiveness and are more vulnerable.

Is it my fault?

Those pesky stormy periods, when it often feels as if "the child changed," can obviously be very worrisome for parents. Suddenly the happy and calm little baby turns into a whiny and angry kid who wants to do everything the opposite way and who is not satisfied, no matter what you do. Who sleeps restlessly and eats poorly, who leaves behind all their good old ways. Who might behave badly, lie down on the floor at the store and scream, or spit on old ladies, or yell profanities.

We do not recognize our child. Instead of being proud and getting compliments and appreciation from others, we get bitter comments and raised eyebrows. Sometimes we even feel thoroughly ashamed.

And what do we as parents do? Obviously, we feel perplexed. We alternate between being strict and regretting our rigor afterwards. Sometimes we manage to stay calm and patient. Sometimes we are just sad and feel like crying. We roar, nag, punish, reward, and cry alternately. In other words, we try all methods and generally do not feel pleased with any of them. And least of all with ourselves.

All good plans and intentions about being calm and consistent fall flat and we feel like failed parents tormented by a guilty conscience. We blame ourselves—we must have made a mistake since he has become such a pain. Have I been too lenient, too strict, too present, or too absent? I, who dreamed about becoming an understanding, mature, and wise parent, and here I am yelling, punishing, threatening, and behaving like a three-year-old myself. What have I done wrong?

But it is not about the child being a failure in any way, and he or she has not been fundamentally transformed either. We have not failed in parenting nor have we failed as parents.

The fact that the child enters a "squabble" now and then is a completely natural and necessary development. Just when the child is about to take a big leap in his development, life becomes chaotic. Then the child is whiny, defiant, angry, and impatient, but basically this is something positive. And it will pass. After each period of defiance comes a quieter time, when the child stops and uses his newly learned skills in order to eventually get into a new period of chaos and development.

The child makes you the parent you are

It is not only the child who goes through his intense developmental periods – we parents do too. But the child goes ahead and leads the way, and we may as well keep up.

16

Those who have more than one child know that we are not the same with all our children. Each child requires different things of us, so this makes us address him or her differently too. If we get a very sensitive and cautious child, we become, for example, overprotective. The next child might perhaps be lively and cocky. If we were overprotective with that child, we would realize that it is not needed.

We, as parents of the child – often without even thinking about it – meet the child halfway. We respond accordingly with how the child is as a person. We address a quiet child calmly, we get annoyed with a whiny child, and yell more quickly at an angry child. This results in not always treating all siblings equally, and often seems unreasonable. This is why we can say that children in the same family have different childhoods. But of course, the way in which we respond to our children also depends on how we are as people.

Nor can we do what others do. Some parents can, for example, go away for a whole weekend when the baby is just a year old. For others, it feels inconceivable to leave the child even at age three. It does not depend on how the parents are, but on how the child is. It is we as parents who best know the child and we know when he is mature. Therefore, it is not a good idea for outsiders to comment on when the child should be left with a babysitter, when to stop breastfeeding, when to start daycare, when they should sleep on their own, and so on.

There is no clear answer to why we become so different in our personalities. But most scientists agree that it depends both on genes and the environment.

We are born with different temperaments, and the environment can influence our behavior, or for example, a disease we catch, placement among siblings, and other external events. Starting school, changing grades, or moving are all examples of other external events that may have an impact, as well as the parents separating, or a death of a family member or friend.

Pondering and processing around the clock

We think a lot during each developmental period. Even the youngest take in, store, and process all that they experience, but in a more subconscious way. We ponder and reflect on the big questions in life. Thoughts about death are common, as are thoughts on where we come from and where we are going and why we live. We think about what kind of a person we will become. During each defiance age, we practice being able to be alone and we need to do it.

In troubled times we also dream more; this is something that has been discovered when people have been studied in sleep laboratories. It is as if we do not have time for all of our thoughts during the day so we need the night to help us out. Sleep problems are extremely common in defiance periods. Many people, both children and adults, tend to have nightmares then. Nightmares fulfill a function: they help us to process difficult thoughts and events in order to move on. Night terrors – when the baby wakes up and screams and is completely inaccessible – are also common, especially when the child is between one and two years old, and at about four years of age. It is similar to sleepwalking. Both night terrors and sleepwalking are hereditary.

There are no simple solutions

When you are in the midst of a difficult period, when there is a conflict from morning to evening about almost everything, you can get completely exhausted. Then it is not surprising if you long for a method, a way of being that kind of a parent who makes it all calmer and better functioning.

In recent years there has been an abundance of parenting support programs in the U.S. designed to help us parents with our defiant child. We see various nanny programs on television. We read about fast-working solutions that will bring order by setting limits, or for example, by relegating children to the corner.

But there are really no simple solutions, no shortcuts, and there are no tricks that suit everyone. Every child and every parent is different. The five-minute method, for example, which is used to get children to fall asleep more easily, fits some children and parents, but far from all. We have to get through these tough times and comfort ourselves with the fact that the defiance periods are necessary and that in their essence they are positive. And moreover, they pass. What usually helps is talking to other parents who have children in the same age group. It is nice to share and hear about others' struggles, especially if you (like most people) think that it is just your child who is so difficult and you who are so unsuccessful.

Perhaps you may even laugh about it together.

HERE, THERE IS HELP

If you feel that you actually cannot handle the problem alone, contact the Children's Health Center and ask to speak to a children's health psychologist or contact a child psychiatry group or a private child psychologist.

Defiance. Open or bold resistance or disregard to an opposing force or authority.
Defiant. Marked by resistance or bold opposition to authority; challenging.
Obstinate age. A period in the development of children around the age of three when they begin to assert their independence and self-will.

BONNIER'S SWEDISH DICTIONARY

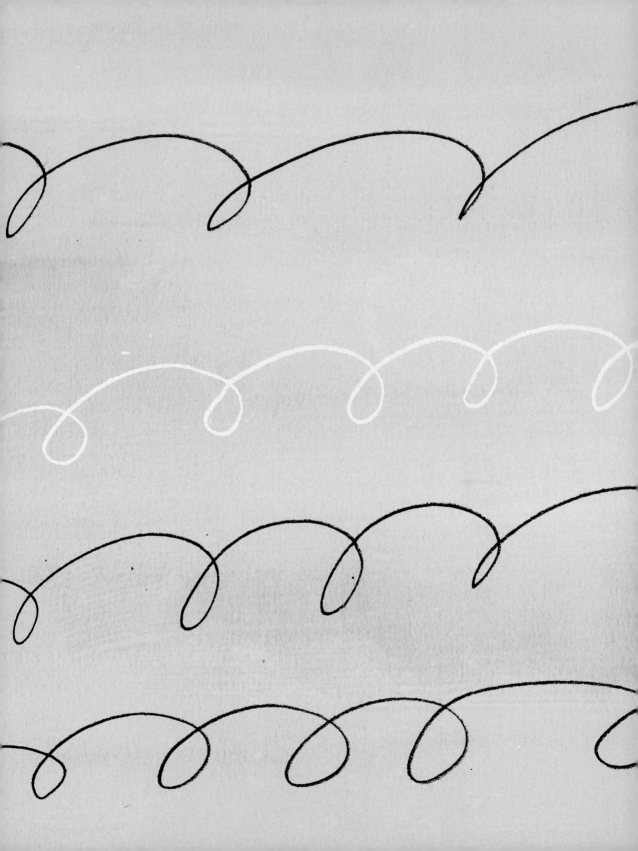

7

Seven leaps during the first year

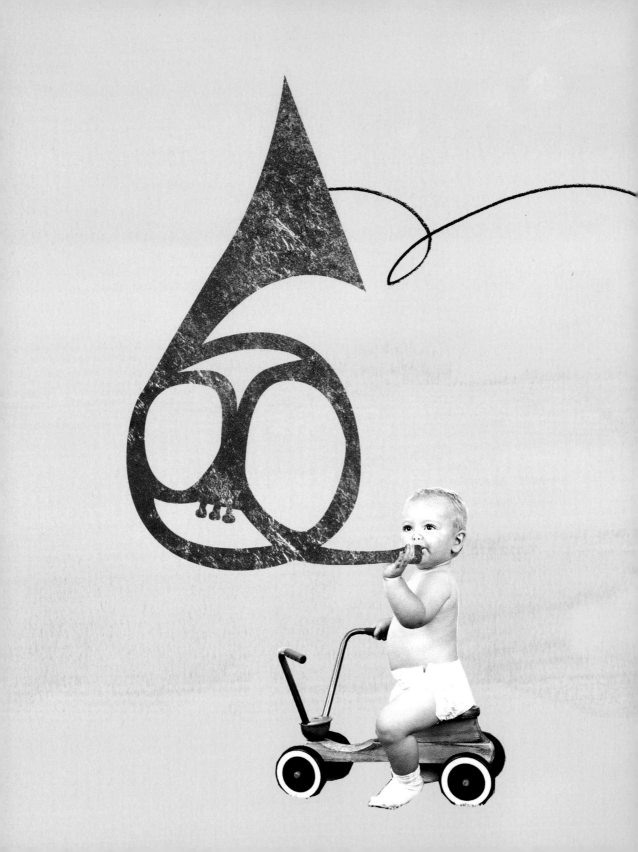

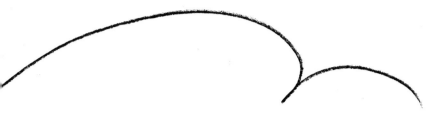

THE FIRST YEAR IS A busy year as the child evolves in both body and soul, more than in any other period in life.

The physical development we all already know about. The child learns how to lift its head, how to turn, grasp, sit, crawl, stand, and maybe walk at about the same age and usually in the same order.

The child also develops mentally according to a certain pattern. Researchers found that infants go through no less than seven important mental developmental leaps in their first year.

What is interesting is that even the mental development occurs at almost the same age for different children. Children go through all of these seven stages of development, but some leaps can pass almost unnoticed for some of them. Most parents become both nonplussed and anxious when the child changes. They do not really recognize their child and wonder what is wrong and often accuse themselves. Have I spoiled my child? Is he insecure? Does she not feel good? They might go to the doctor or the Child's Health Center to ask if there is something wrong with the child.

Development is not a malfunction, but an intense period of changes makes life more challenging and it can be unsettling for both parents and the child. But this doesn't mean anything is wrong.

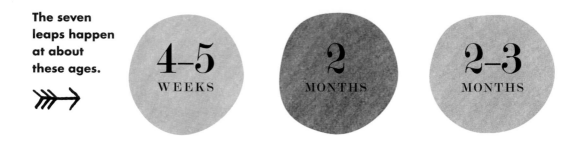

Before each developmental leap, the child becomes more demanding and wants more attention than usual. The clingy period preceding each leap usually comes weeks prior. When such a period is over, the child is happier, more peaceful, and more independent than before.

All the leaps consist of three phases

Every developmental leap has three stages or phases:

PREPARING PHASE. When the child requires extra attention and is generally difficult. They often take a few steps back in their development. The parents do not recognize their child and the child does not recognize himself and therefore becomes frustrated. The child sleeps and eats less, screams more, and is more clingy and whiny. He is also shy and quieter than before.

It is as if the child knows he will soon know something he is still not yet able to know. This is why the child becomes so impatient.

DEVELOPING PHASE. Now comes the actual developmental stage, which varies from time to time.

ENDING PHASE. Each leap ends with a quiet phase when the child is happier and more independent than before. The child rests after the difficult developing phase and gathers strength for the following leap.

Both the child and the parents enjoy his new skills.

24

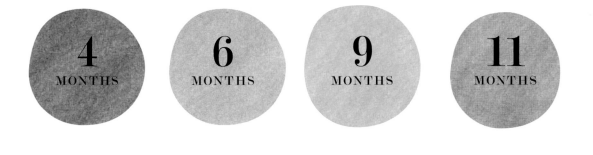

Developmental leaps

THE FIRST LEAP comes at about four to five weeks old, when the child goes through several important physical changes. For instance, the child starts to cry real tears, is able to focus his eyes, and breathes more regularly. He vomits and belches less frequently and can stay awake for longer periods.

You can help your baby by rocking, carrying, hugging, caressing, and breastfeeding him.

THE SECOND LEAP is when the child is about two months old. Then she discovers her fingers and toes, is able to see shadows, light, darkness, and patterns. There are many new impressions that the child needs to get used to, and a safe and familiar environment is needed. Therefore, the child becomes unusually needy for mommy and daddy and is also loud and demanding. Sensitive children cry more than before.

You can help your child by looking at things together. Let her lie without socks so that she can play with her toes. Take a bath together. Put some music on and dance with your baby. Try the "pull up game" when the

Before each leap the child suffers similar symptoms:

- Screams more often
- Wants more physical contact and more attention
- Eats less
- Sleeps poorly
- Is shyer and clingier than usual
- Sucks more

About Helga,
six months old

She just screams and kicks all day long. She also started waking up at night again. She does not know how to occupy herself at all. This is very difficult, for example if we go out she does not want to ride in the stroller, she just screams. I cannot take it anymore, I do not have anyone to leave her with either. I feel like a failure as a mother.

child can hold her head steady. A mobile phone, a music box, or a beautiful fabric next to the bed is exciting. Fold down the baby stroller canopy when walking and place the bed by the window so that the baby can see light and shadows, moving leaves or clouds, or raindrops on the window.

THE THIRD LEAP is at about two to three months old. Now the child often takes a step back. If she has been able to be entertained on her own before, she no longer can. The child becomes clingy and needy for mom and dad. The baby's movements become smoother. She learns nuances. The child may perceive changes in vision, hearing, taste, and smell impressions. She can also track things with her eyes, get an overview of a room, and recognize sounds in a more nuanced way then before. The baby may try to make different sounds. You can help the child by "talking" to her in different ways: in a loud voice or whispering, by gargling, whistling, smacking, and so on. Or you can let you child feel different surfaces, such as fur, wood, plastic, and silk.

THE FOURTH LEAP occurs when the baby is about four months old. Then she learns to do several things. The child can grasp a rattle, but also shake it, turn it over, look at it, and put it in her mouth. The baby discovers that things exist even though they are not visible, and playing peekaboo is fun. The child explores things with her hands. Making sounds is also interesting and now the child might begin to practice imitating sounds similar to those of mom and dad.

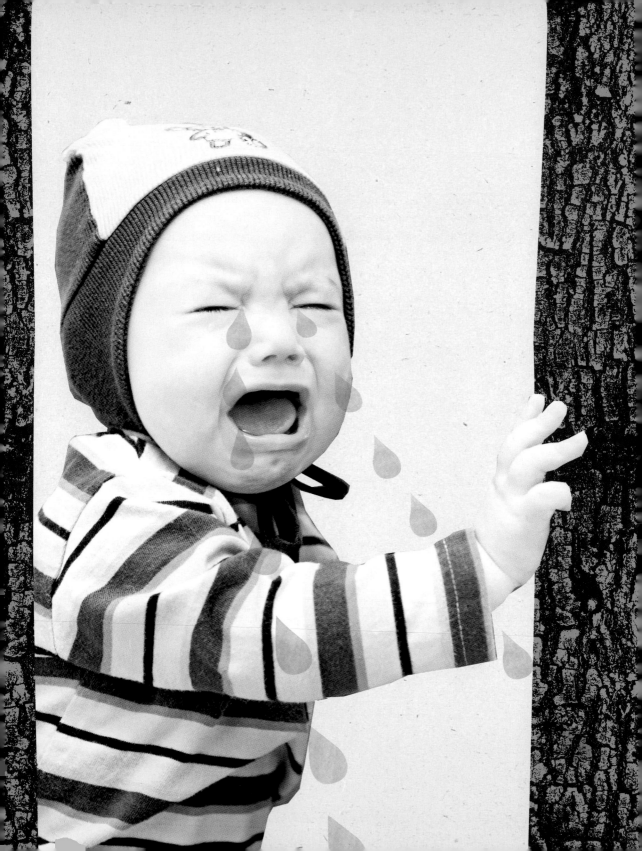

About Amanda,
seven months old

I really love her, but recently she has become so annoying. Previously she was so kind and almost always happy. She sleeps at night, but every day she wakes up early and I breastfeed her. Afterwards she is very pleased and happy. But after an hour and a half, she becomes cranky and tired. She gets fed and then she just wants to sleep, but it is so difficult. The only one who makes her fall asleep is the babysitter, but first, when you put her there it is almost like sticking a knife into her. And after a while she falls asleep anyway.

Motor development is great. You can help your child by looking at picture books, playing peek-a-boo, singing, playing music, and tumbling around with the baby.

THE FIFTH LEAP is at about six months old. It is called the relational leap because now the child starts to put himself in relation to others. The child learns that he is very small and that the world is very big. If mom and dad go into another room they "disappear." Therefore it obviously feels scary and therefore the child preferably wants to be close to the parents. The child becomes more shy and can have difficulties in falling asleep and sleeping peacefully. They can also have nightmares.

You can help your child by showing that you are not abandoning him and letting him get used to new situations calmly. It is time for games, such as peekaboo, rigmaroles, and building towers that the child gets to knock over.

THE SIXTH LEAP occurs when the child is around nine months old. Now, the child is clingier than ever, sleeps poorly, loses its appetite, and suffers mood changes. He can become whiny and angry and quite demanding. Now, the greatest and most important leap of the first year takes place. It is a time when parents often do not recognize their child. The happy and calm child can become very difficult.

You can read about this developmental leap in the next chapter of the book.

THE SEVENTH LEAP, the last in the first year of life, occurs at about eleven months of age. A few weeks previous to that, the child becomes listless, clingy, and less vivid than before. This leap implies that the child learns that order is important. First you get undressed, and then you bathe. The child becomes more aware of his actions. If you eat the cake, then it is gone. If you push the tower, the blocks fall.

About Albin, eight months old

My son has changed from being a hassle-free and happy child. He has been a little ray of sunshine, happy and satisfied with life. Now he whines and squeals all day long. Nothing is good, except for when he is being carried. He can scream for half an hour before falling asleep. He is also anxious at night. I have no idea why and what I have done wrong.

The baby exercises his body all the time by climbing, crawling, throwing balls, and so forth. It also trains to start eating on his own and maybe to stand and walk.

You can help your child by giving him new, exciting toys, like a large, light ball and a simple puzzle.

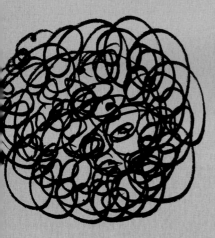

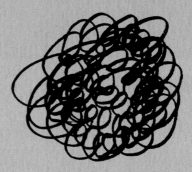

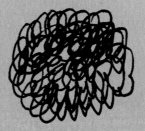

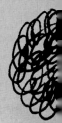
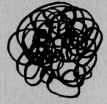

Nine months old – time for passion

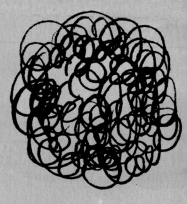

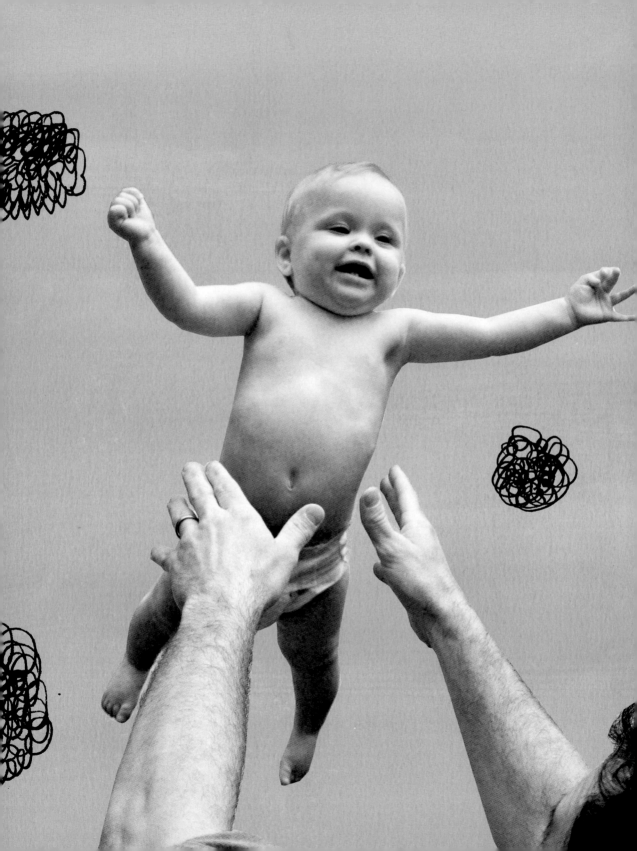

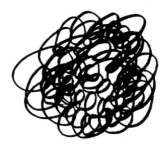

WHEN THE CHILD IS ABOUT nine months old, suddenly there are even more things happening in her development. This is partly connected with the child learning to get around and then becoming more independent. It is great but also scary. Therefore, in this age, the child becomes more clingy and needy for mom and dad. The child is also often angry and whiny.

For the parents, the transformation from calm and happy to whiny and angry can be worrying, but it is a completely natural part of development. Obviously, this change rarely comes exactly at nine months; it can come a little before or a little after.

Now, something important happens in the life of the child. The baby, who earlier laid where she laid or sat where you seated her, learns to go where she wants by crawling (or slithering, sitting on her buttocks and jumping forward).

For us parents, the child's first steps usually feel like a big milestone. But actually, it is an even greater event in the child's life to learn to crawl, because this is the first time she can move around. Walking is just another way. But being able to get to the coveted toy or to access something that looks exciting in order to investigate it is a revolution in life.

Before the child learns to crawl, she often becomes whiny and dissatisfied. She wants so badly to be able to do it, but cannot. She

**About Rosa,
nine months old**

My second daughter was always sweet, quiet, and happy, she basically never cried. Now, at nine moths old, she is suddenly horribly cranky. She gets mad when she is unable or not allowed to do something.

has a goal but cannot quite reach it. This creates great frustration. Even children who previously have been mild and "nice" can become grumpy and only want to be in mom's or dad's arms. Only the parents can help, the child seems to think.

When the child suddenly is different, parents are often anxious and a little nonplussed. What happened? I do not recognize my child. She has always has been so calm and happy. And then the usual question: What have I done wrong? But nothing is wrong, neither with the parents nor with the child. This is just a natural part of development.

Now we require more of the child

When the "nice" child becomes difficult, parents often get annoyed. It is good for us to do so. We can say that in this way we help the child in his development.

We convey to the child that now they have to learn to crawl and get what they want on their own. Now, whining is not enough, I do not have time for that. I will not help you. When we become annoyed we kind of push the baby out from the nest, much like birds do. We often do this for the first time when the baby is about nine months old. And this is just right and not something we should feel guilty for.

We are also starting to talk to the child in a different way than before. Before, we just lifted the baby away if he did something dangerous. Now we also exhort. Doing so is part of letting the child grow and become more self-dependent.

Now when the child can move around, it becomes very clear that mom and dad are two separate beings, and not "two in one" like during pregnancy.

34

The child can even crawl into another room. This is why we can call the nine-month mark the second cut of the umbilical cord.

Then, we parents often take our thoughts back to the first cutting of the umbilical cord, when the child was born. Many people start thinking more about the birth now, and it is not a coincidence. Becoming a parent is a big change and it does not happen as if by magic at birth. It takes nine months for the child to stop growing in the stomach and we also grow as parents. Then it takes at least another nine months before we switch over to being a parent. The developmental period at nine months is thus an important maturation period for both the child and the parents.

Now, it is common that the child has problems with sleeping, and it can become even more difficult with children who have a history of sleeping difficulties. The child is woken up by dreams because he needs to make sure you are still there, now when he is moving away from you. Almost all children do this. The fact that the child has difficulties falling asleep and is waking up at night can be incredibly difficult for the parents—sometimes it can feel like you cannot take it anymore, that you will not survive. Then it is good to remind yourself that it will pass and that it is not your fault that the child is not sleeping.

There are no rules for coping with sleep difficulties. However, there are different tricks to try out: carrying the child, letting him fall asleep to music, going in the stroller, putting the baby on your stomach or on your lap, letting the vacuum cleaner drone in the next room. It may be

About Leo, almost nine months old

He has not yet learned to crawl. But I think he has the feeling that he will soon be able to. He has always been so quiet and "nice" and now he is cranky and impatient. You can really see how much he longs to be able to get around. He is so frustrated over not being able to crawl yet. As a parent you feel helpless. You cannot teach him to crawl.

About Irju, nine and a half months old

My son is wonderful and I love him very much, but occasionally he gets on my nerves. He likes to bang on things and we have told him that the TV and the aquarium are absolutely forbidden to bang on. We tried to say no calmly, removing him, or becoming upset and saying no in a harsher way. He thinks it is great fun when we get angry and then he crawls back again and bangs even harder. In the end, I cannot take it anymore and get enraged and tear him away from there. Then he gets really sad and I get the worst anxiety for being so angry.

helpful to have your child in your bed in your bedroom, if you can manage to sleep like this. It can be equally right to let him lie in his own bed. Sometimes it can be helpful for the child to be pushed away from mom and dad. So there is no right way, no magic formula. Here we must use trial and error. In a period of sleep problems, it is wise to ignore all the principles and make it easy for ourselves. For example, allowing the child to fall asleep on the couch with the TV on.

There are also various sleep-training methods. The most common is the so-called five-minute method. It is based on teaching the child to fall asleep and fall back to sleep on its own. You put the baby in his own bed and go out and leave the door slightly ajar. If the baby cries, you wait for a couple of minutes and then go in and check on the baby, but without lifting or comforting him; you just show it that you are there. Then you leave the room again and continue like this until the child falls asleep. Many children scream and object for half an hour, but a week later they have learned to fall asleep on their own. It is a method that suits some children and some parents. Those who like the method say that the child will become calmer and feel safer. It will gain confidence as he learns to fall asleep and fall back to sleep. The child also becomes happier and healthier because he gets enough sleep. For other parents, this method does not work at all. They think it is cruel and difficult to let the child scream and consider the method as a return to authoritarian upbringing. For the most part, the reaction of the child is what determines if the five-minute method is suitable or not. There are few parents who are capable of implementing this method if the child reacts with despair. Then, it seems easier to deal with the child being upset.

36

Love for the parents

At nine months old the child is extremely enamored with his parents and especially with the one who accounts for the daily care. He knows that mom is mom and that she is the only one, and this is an important insight. The fact that the mother is the one who, during this period, is subject to an impetuous passion, obviously depends on that the mother is the one who has lived closest to the child during pregnancy and after birth, and the fact that it has always been mom who provides the food. But the more time the child spends with Dad, the more he becomes attached to him.

Children can show their love in different ways. Many are very physical. They chew on their mother, give her true love bites, they seem to want to eat her. Or they cling to her and pinch her, suck on her, and pull her hair. Others may sit glued to the parent and will not let go even for brief periods. They might yell if anyone even comes close. There are children who also show their love in a quieter way. Babies, just like adults, have different temperaments and express themselves differently. During this intense love period, the child practices love expressions and rules. This is a preparation for the passions that may come later in life—for example, at age three to four at age six, in adolescence, and later. Being so loved and worshipped as a parent is wonderful, but also tough. Sometimes, all this love and clinginess is difficult to bear. Often we do not even think that it is about love, but we just feel tired and irritable. It is hard even for the other parent, who wants to help to relieve, but is not "allowed." Felling rejected can also be difficult. But this clingy period passes and soon the other parent is good enough too.

About William, nine months old

He never gets enough! He clings on to me day and night, no one else may take him. When his dad tries to take him he screams. Sometimes he bites me so hard with his teeth that it hurts. I do not know what to do. I am about to start working and Dad is going to take over. I do not know how it will turn out.

About Anja, nine months old

Anja owns me, for some time now she has totally ruled over me. If she is allowed, she constantly climbs and clings on me, from morning to evening. She pinches and bites me on my neck and arms. She is passionately in love with me. It is almost as if she is a drug addict who simply must have her drug, and the drug is me. It is flattering, but also hard because only I will do. Unfortunately, her father has to work long hours during the week and then it is mostly on me. But on weekends he devotes a lot of time to her and then she accepts him and bonds with him too. The daddy-ness obviously grows the more time they spend together. But the mummy-ness is completely dominant.

After a while, a toddler always accepts the one who gives him love and time. At this stage of development, most children can also show a furious rage and this forms part of the great passion. By being "impossible," the child tests if the love is real. It is just the ones who we truly love we dare to defy. Once the baby feels secure in his love, he can sometimes become really difficult. Thus, the baby needs this anger in order to grow and develop. For the parents, this transformation the child goes through – from being calm and happy to whiny and angry – is often enigmatic and almost scary. One wonders where is the child one had before, and wonders if this is going to last forever. Then it can feel good to realize that almost all children go through such a transformation when they are about nine months old. The child must become this "awkward" to be able to develop further.

Tumultuous period

Since nine months old is a major developmental age, it is often said that this is not a good time for big changes. During this time, it may for example be tough to leave the child with strangers. How strongly the baby reacts varies; therefore it is important to pay attention to the child's response.

If at this age, the father takes over at home, it is important that the father and the child already have established a close relationship before. Then, the switch between mom and dad usually happens smoothly. It may also be helpful if the mother does not completely stop breastfeeding when she starts working, since too many changes at this time can be hard on the baby.

But if the changes need to be done, then it is also okay. Children are good at compensating. They can, for example, use the night to be close to mom, if she starts working when the child is nine months old.

THINGS TO CONSIDER

→ The child often becomes very impatient and frustrated just before he learns to crawl.

→ Now the "second cut of the umbilical cord" happens: the child becomes more independent.

→ It is common that the child is passionately in love with his parents. He is clingy, mostly to the one who accounts for the daily care.

→ Clinginess and the great love may be annoying. But the more you affirm the clinginess the faster it will pass. Long playing and clinging moments lead to greater serenity.

→ Naturally, one sometimes gets angry and irritated with the child who loves intensely and very tangibly. We certainly have the right to put a stop to hard pinches and sharp teeth. Then the child learns that a good and vivid relationship is a little bit less vigorous. By keeping the child at a little distance we help him to liberate himself.

→ For those who currently feel rejected: in the long run the child always accepts the one who loves him and gives him time.

→ Anger and whininess form part of the child's great love. It is normal for the child to be transformed from a sunshine to a yeller now.

→ As a parent, we are now the child's first guide. This means that we must affirm his love but also put a stop to it.

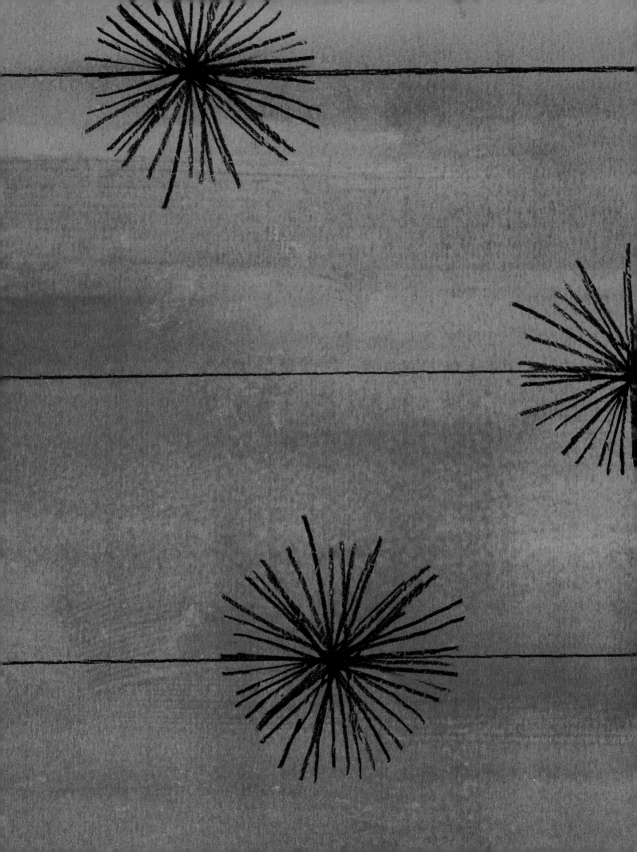

2

Two years old – period of frontal collisions

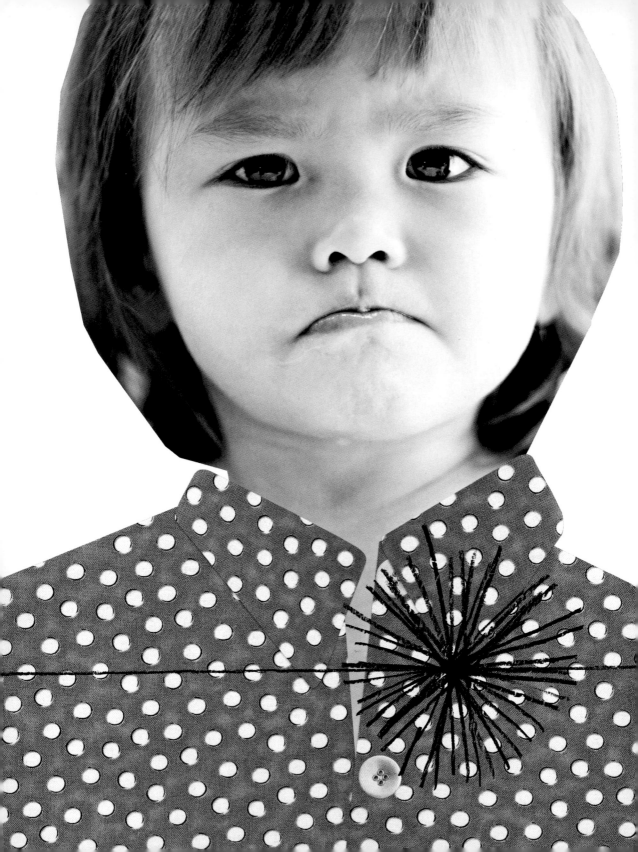

STUDIES HAVE SHOWN that minor conflicts between two to three year-olds and their parents occur every three minutes, and major conflicts three to four times per hour.

The fact that there are so many conflicts now is not because there is something wrong with the child or because we have failed with the upbringing, which is always very easy to believe as a parent.

Living with a defiant two-year-old can be very tiring; sometimes it is so hard that we almost cannot stand it. This is normal and is not because we are bad parents. When the child refuses to put on the warm overalls though the temperature is below zero and the train leaves in ten minutes, or when he lies down on the floor in the store screaming his heart out and everyone stares, it can be difficult to stay calm and also to be consistent. We alternate in rapid successions between bribes, rage, and attempts at persuasion. But we can actually also endure it. Since we have to get through it, we actually do. When we are in the midst of misery, it feels as if it will go on forever. But one day it calms down, and the period of perturbation is over for this time. But there will be other developmental periods. One reason for why the two to three-year-old age range is filled with conflicts is because "the honeymoon

About Paul, two and a half years old

We were abroad and stayed at a hotel this summer. Every evening we ate dinner in the restaurant, so it was necessary to dress well. Paul hates wearing formal wear and we had endless conflicts. But then we began to play the "end-of-it" game. He got to choose which one of three outfits I would wear. Then I told him which outfit I did not want. And then he said triumphantly "That's the end of it, no hassle Mom." Then, I would have to wear that outfit. And then it was the other way around. This became a game he looked forward to the whole day. We have continued to play it at home as well, and thus we avoid all the fuss about clothes.

is now over." Earlier, the child had been the total center of mom and dad's life; he had been quite certain that he has governed the world, including everyone in the family. Now this time is over. The child realizes that there are different wills: the wills of the parents and also of others. Before, we had fewer expectations of the child understanding and doing as we want. We certainly have admonished the child but we have not expected him to obey. Now, we suddenly have completely different demands of the child; he should preferably both understand and obey. For the child, this is a shock. But the stubborn two-year-old will not give up. Why would he? He fights with full force to get his way. The child is not convinced by the parent's arguments and does not obey, but as parents we still keep correcting the child.

"I can do it myself"

Another major cause of conflicts is that now the child knows how to do many things that he could not do before. He can get things on his own, he can get food and eat on his own. He can dress fairly well on his own and climb in and out of the stroller and walk next to it on his own. Many two to three year-olds are already sitting in front of the computer. "I can myself" becomes like a battle-cry that permeates most of the daily life. The child is full of confidence and optimism. He believes he can cope with everything. The two to three-year-old is often very helpful and happy to help out in the kitchen or with cleaning. It can help when the laundry is being sorted and with cleaning or arranging shoes by hallway entrance. It might not be perfect and it does not happen fast, but it is great to be able to do it "by myself."

Doing the same thing many times is also typical at this age. Up and down the stairs twenty-five times, opening and closing doors, putting together the same puzzle. And woe to those who do not want to do as the child pleases. The child would love to take command of the surroundings and allocate tasks. "You do this and you do that," or "now I am going to sit here and then I will . . ." Self-confidence grows. And then when mom or dad tries to limit their freedom by saying stop, it is clear that the child feels violated and violent conflicts arise.

Or, the child tries to cope with something with all his might, but fails. This also feels like a violation and usually leads to a powerful outburst. If "I can myself" is one mantra, then the other one is "no." With a definite no, the child can control their environment, and show their power. Of course she will say no, almost always automatically and very fast. There may even be a no although the child wants a yes. It can become a fixed idea; the child can get "stuck" in saying no, as one father said.

The conflicts may involve almost anything. A power struggle at the dinner table is common. Breaking up is hard and there may be violent outbursts when it is time to go to daycare – and when it is time to go

> **About**
> **Tindra, two years**
> **and eight months old**
>
> She was at the movies for the first time. Actually, she was probably too small, but she came along because we went with her older siblings. However, she was the one who had the greatest experience. She was completely blissful and when the movie was over, everybody started to go home and they began cleaning the salon, and she waited for "more movies." Our persuasion attempts were useless. Eventually we had to carry her out, while she was desperately screaming for more movies, to the car without any warm clothing in freezing weather.

**About Axel,
two years and nine
months old**

Everyone thinks of our son as a pain. We get a lot of criticism and it makes me feel as if I cannot take care of my child. But to us, he is the most beautiful thing there is.

home. Clothing and sleep are other common causes of conflict. All of us who have a defiant two-year-old ponder over how to handle these conflicts. She is both small and big – one minute she is cocky, and another minute she is small and mumsy and dadsy. She understands a whole lot, but maybe not as much as we think and above all not when she is at her angriest.

First, probably no parent is capable of having only one way of being. We always strive to keep our principles in raising children and being consistent, but we cannot always manage it, otherwise we would not be human. Sometimes we are so challenged that we ourselves become like three-year-olds and behave more or less like the child. If we are tired and stressed for example, then we can "take" fewer fights than if we were alert and rested. Being at home or away also affects our reactions.

Second, it would not be good if we would only have one way of being. It is important for the child's development in the future to learn that one can and may become angry and lose one's temper sometimes. I, as well as mom and dad, can be that way.

Dare to be angry

Many parents are unaccustomed to speaking up and asserting themselves. We have heard that we should speak calmly with our child, and we become distraught and feel guilty when the calm conversation instead becomes a violent conflict where we yell like fools and end up using pure strength to force

**About Matt,
three years old**

At daycare, now and then he shows his temper, but he does not have any outbursts similar to those he has here at home.

46

the child. We wonder if we inhibited and repressed our child, if we harmed it for life. But putting a stop to a child who behaves badly is not to inhibit or subdue; it is to help the child. Even if the child is only two years old, we can and should talk to him after the fight.

About Balder, two years old

What is it with our two-year-old? He has become quite impossible. If he does not get his way though, he screams and his whole face turns red, he begins flailing his arms, kicking and hitting. I feel totally helpless and cry every night.

Not right afterwards, but maybe later or the following day. Often we apologize almost automatically when we become very angry. We should of course do that, if we feel that there is a reason for us to apologize. But if we have been rightfully angry, if there was a reason for our anger, we should not apologize.

A really strong outburst often ends with the child being upset and crying. He understood that he did something wrong and then we parents feel even more guilty. But the outburst is usually not over until the tears come. Only when the child has understood that the parent is serious about their opposition. If we do not stop, the child might feel that we abandoned him. Sometimes we have to carry a shouting and kicking kid. And we must stop the child who bites and hits Dad or another child.

If we parents would give up and behave just as the child pleases, the child's development would be stunted. By demanding things from the children, we actually help them to move forward. The personality and temperament of the child affect our behavior towards them. If we have an unusually stubborn and willful child, it requires an unusual amount of firmness from us parents. Then, there will also be an unusual amount of nagging and conflicts at home. Obviously, our own temperament also affects our behavior towards the child. But if we have a child who is sensitive and fragile, and who would rather resort to crying

47

About Fanny, three years old

She has always been strong-willed, but now she contradicts everything. There is a battle about absolutely everything: shoes, clothes, when to go home from daycare, what to do and what not to do. She is her worst towards me. With her father, she is much more reasonable. I think a lot about the reason for this and what I have done wrong.

than screaming, our behavior is obviously different, more cautious. Therefore, it may happen that we treat siblings differently.

We can strive for justice, but often, children cannot be treated equally. A certain child needs more and another needs less firmness. We could say that different children require different things from us. We cannot always be the same. Therefore, we become different parents to different children and during such periods, this is clearly visible. Giving the child resistance in everything is not a good thing. We have to choose our conflicts in order not to become exhausted. Some things we need to battle for, such as taking medication and brushing teeth. And of course, vital things such as not crossing the street alone and not being alone in the bathroom while bathing. But perhaps it is not necessary to argue about things such as whether the child should wear the red or the yellow dress today, or that he must finish eating the potatoes he said he wanted.

One tip is to not fuss unnecessarily about food, sleep, pee, and poo at these ages. It does not mean that the child will be allowed to eat lasagna or meatballs every day, or that she may go to bed when she feels like it, or pee on the carpet. But do not force your child to eat all of her food or to sit on the potty. Such action of enforcement may at its worst lead to problems later on. It is easy to create a bad "fuss habit." When a child defies us a lot, we as parents end up giving the child resistance all the time. Then it is wise to stop and reflect. What is really important to fight about? And then ignore some of the trouble. Consistency is not so important during these periods of defiance. Now, the child usually knows the rules. It is therefore okay if we sacrifice some of the principles for a while.

Putting your foot down

There are four reasons for why we have to put a stop to the child. Reason 1 and reason 2 are obvious for most, but reasons 3 and 4 are far from it. They may even feel challenging.

1. FOR THE CHILD TO BE PROTECTED. For example, from getting hurt in traffic or from ingesting something dangerous.

2. FOR THE CHILD TO FEEL GOOD. She must have nutritious food, not get cavities, get enough sleep, and not be cold or get wet. We as parents are the ones who need to teach our children the everyday order of things, and this can practically turn everyday life into a power struggle from morning to night.

3. FOR THE CHILD TO BECOME A SOCIAL BEING. She needs to be able to live and function with others, not only at home but also out in society. A child who always gets what it wants becomes unbearable to live with. If the child does not have any limits, she will not be liked by other children or adults. She will get a negative response from others and become isolated.

4. BECAUSE THE CHILD NEEDS RESISTANCE. Having conflicts with other people is a necessary and inevitable part of growth and maturation. Conflicts are needed for the child to develop into an independent individual who is aware of its own desires and needs and who can take other people's desires and needs into account. And you can often see the child feeling satisfied after a battled conflict.

About Alva, two years old

Oftentimes not a whole lot is needed for a difficult situation to change. Anger may come and go quickly. Yesterday at daycare, she was lying on the floor crying because she did not want to get dressed and go home. Then she saw a photo of herself on the wall and in the middle of a scream she stopped abruptly, giggled and said, "Look, there's Alva."

49

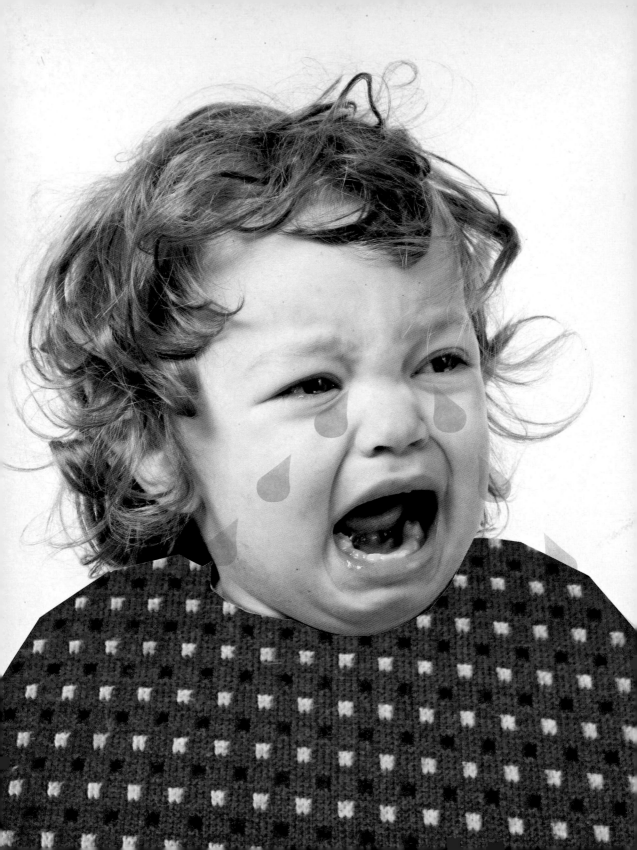

There is always a reason

As a parent of a two-year-old, we often wonder why the child defies when we believe that there is nothing to have caused it. But there is always a cause; it is just that mom and dad may not always understand it. And a two to three-year-old does not have enough language to be able to explain it. Suddenly, the child does not want to eat a certain kind of food, even though it always liked that particular food. Perhaps it is because the food in its appearance reminds the child of a food it once had and then felt sick of. Children make connections that we adults do not always understand. For the child it is logical, but for the parents it is illogical.

One day, the child refuses to bathe in the tub, but it has loved to bathe ever since it was a baby. Mom and dad do not get it. Nothing awful has happened in the tub. But the child has its reasons. It might have seen how the water from the tub is lost in a whirlpool and thought "What if I disappear in the same way?" The child has seen the whirlpool many times before, but only now can the child draw conclusions. Hence, the sudden and inexplicable terror of the tub.

Similarly, the child may become frightened of the toilet and does not dare to sit on it anymore. The child has suffered a sudden insight and sees things from a new perspective. And therefore the child's behavior changes. Children at this age often have a magical way of thinking. If things are not done in a specific order then everything is "wrong." The

About Jordan, three years old

He can get angry super-fast and it we do not always know why. He gets real outbursts, he screams, kicks and hits. Things fly all over the place. If it is possible, he is left alone until he calms down, and then he comes back on his own. Sometimes, I get to hold him in my arms and then he becomes quiet and sad instead. Other times, I carry away or dress a wriggling and screaming child with more or less violence. My heart hurts and I feel so guilty, but what should I do?

51

child may, for example, become hysterical because dad pours milk before porridge in a bowl.

Sometimes we parents understand the child's reasons, perhaps long afterwards and by chance. However, most often we do not understand them at all, but it usually helps just to know that the child has its reasons.

Defiance – mostly towards the parents

Many parents tell us that the child behaves completely different at home and away. At home, you have a little savage, but to your surprise you hear that the child behaves well at daycare and at grandmother's house. The surrounding people are unsympathetic – what have you got to complain about, she is nothing but kind? This is very common, and this is how it should be. This means that the child is safe with its parents. It dares to behave exactly as it feels. Together with us parents the child dares to show its anger. It knows that we love it even though it is troublesome. Not always for what it does, but for what it is. The fact that the child dares to defy its parents is kind of a declaration of love. A child who feels good is supposed to defy the person or people with whom it feels mostly secure. If the child defies, it should thus be seen as a kind of compliment. And this is why the child can be an angel while away, when mom and dad are not around. At daycare, when the child is getting ready to go out and play, perhaps the two-year-old is nice and cooperates while getting dressed.

But when dad comes to pick the child up, the child gets down on the floor and screams when the clothes are to be put on. Then, when dad comes, the child can finally relax and dare to defy. The vigorous development of the two to three-year-old affects everything, from morning to night. And of course, it also affects sleep. The child

About Sebastian, almost three years old

This entire power struggle is becoming increasingly more difficult. I get so angry and irritated and start to cry. Then, I feel so guilty and feel completely failed as a mother.

may have difficulties falling asleep. In maturation periods, it is almost as if we are losing control over the environment.

Things that used to be obvious are now more or less menacing or chaotic. Therefore, children become more dependent on their parents than before. Then it can be frightening to go to sleep and thus leave the parents. Precisely in such periods, the child needs to have its parents close. If we help it to fall asleep safely by lying next to it, usually the trouble of falling asleep soon passes. If you do not want to lie next to your child until it falls asleep (perhaps because you do not want to fall asleep yourself), maybe the child could be allowed to fall asleep on the couch in the living room for some time, until everything comes down.

Another reason the child has difficulties falling asleep may be as simple as life being so much fun that the child does not want to miss out on anything. Then, calm evening rituals, which are the same every night, may be good. This provides security and the child has time to unwind.

About Svante, three years old

Our son, who used to always fall asleep in his own bed in two minutes and slept there for the rest of the night, has now begun to "fuss." We changed our night routines and we now sit next to him until he falls asleep. But now he wakes up around midnight and forcefully wants to lie in our bed. Then we have tried to take him back to his bed and sit with him until he falls asleep – just like in the evening – but it is impossible. He becomes completely hysterical. Sure, it might be nice to have him in our bed but then it would be the whole night every night. We have lost both our "adult evenings" and nights. We have no time on our own.

Many two to three-year-olds, or perhaps most of them, wake up at night and want to come in to mom and dad's bed. Often, this happens because the child dreams. The day is not enough when life is as intense as in ages two to three. Even nights must be used. Therefore children often dream a lot during a period of development. Terrible nightmares about lions, witches, and ghosts are common. Then it is important not to feel abandoned, to have access to mom and dad's bed. Sleeping next to the parents provides security and fear passes faster. It is great if one is able to sleep with the child in bed. The problem is if a parent sleeps poorly. Sometimes the child falls back to sleep quickly, if one can manage to put him back in his own bed, or one can also sit next to his for a while.

One solution would be to get an adult bed for the child and then go to sleep there with the child. Or one could place a guest bed beside the parental bed, which the child could be gently pushed over to when he comes for a visit. Then there is closeness, but also restful sleep.

THINGS TO CONSIDER

→ The child realizes that there are other wills than just the one of its own.

→ It is not dangerous to be angry with your two-year-old and to show anger. This will not inhibit the child.

→ We can and do not have to be consistent during this particular period.

→ Children need to face resistance in order to develop.

→ Sleep disorders are common and will pass.

→ Choose your battles. Argue about what is important.

→ Distracting the child is often a convenient way out.

USEFUL READING (SEE P. 87)

Pippi Longstocking series (Picture books) by Astrid Lindgren

About Vera, two years old

What an ordeal we have every morning! When I
get to work it is time for a deep sigh and a big cup of
coffee. She wants to have her way with everything. She wants
to choose her clothes on her own. It may turn out crazy. Naturally,
she wants to dress herself. It can take ten minutes to put on a pair of
rain boots. If I try to hurry things up or help her she goes mad. Sometimes
she goes into a deadlock and it ends with her lying on the floor on her belly
crying desperately. Then I have to pick her up, comfort her, ease things,
and start over. You have to be in top shape on your own to cope with this
kind of thing. It is a balancing act not to disturb her integrity too much but
still make things work. Some things she just has to have influence over,
but other things, like brushing her teeth, we get to be in charge of.
Vera's brother was exactly the same at that age, although they
are very different in general. It takes two hours from the time
when we wake up until we are done. She needs all of
this time otherwise the whole day is ruined. My wife
and I trade with drop-off and pick-up. I find it
amazingly nice not to be in such a big rush
in the mornings.

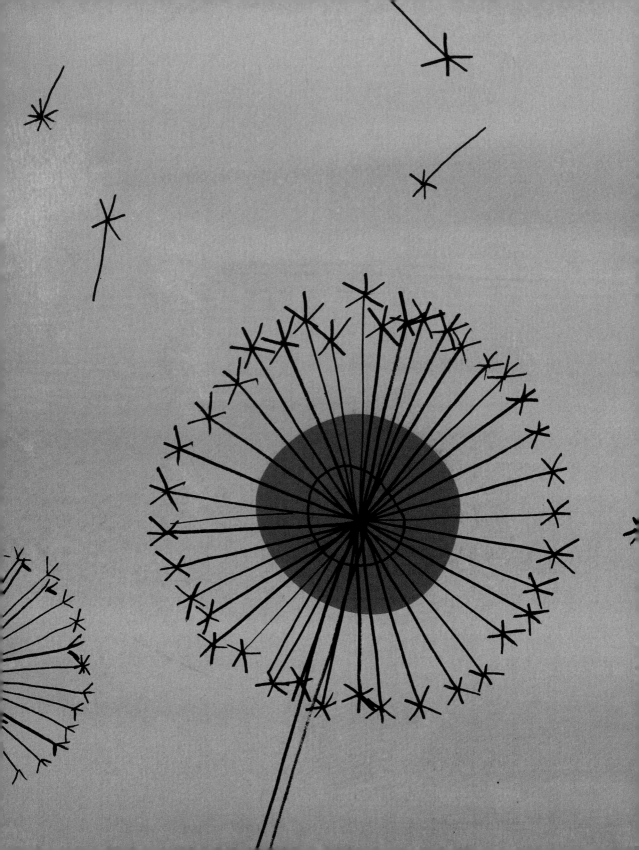

Four years old – the world opens up

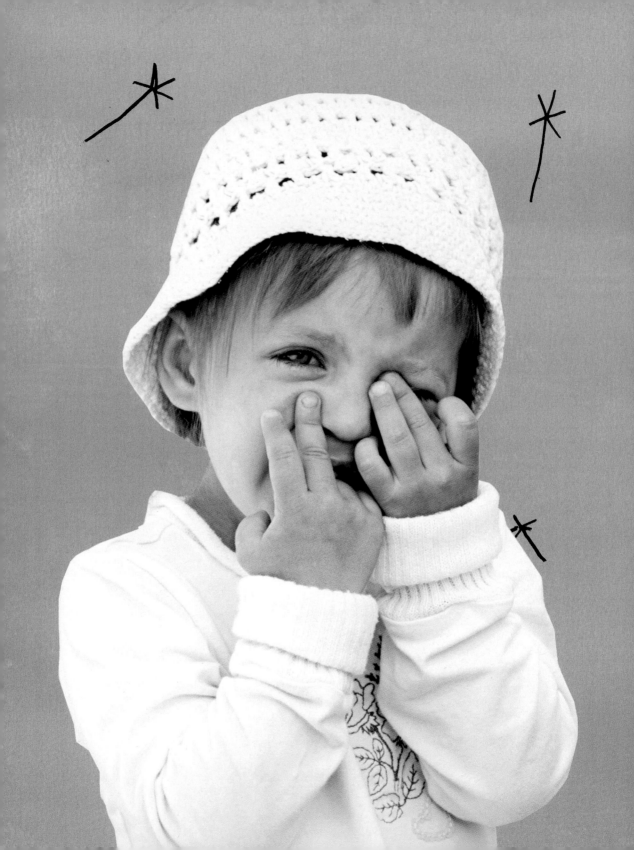

AT AGE FOUR, one of the greatest developmental explosions occurs. In many ways, this is a harmonious time; the child is active and fun, and curiosity and imagination flourish. But as in any other development, there can also be hassles. Seemingly small setbacks can make the child furious. At four years old, there is often a wild struggle for power at home between children and parents. Then it is important to find the right balance. Let your child grow and develop without unnecessary quell and obligation. But also give it the resistance that it needs.

The child is both small and big. It can handle a lot and be big, clever, and plucky. The four-year-old often knows how things should be and likes to tell the parents about it. In one instant, the child may hate both mom and dad and in the next, he wants to crawl into the parent's bed and be really small. At four years of age, most traits are in place, we can guess whether if the child will be a slob or nitpicky, if he will be practical or more theoretical. The child is driven by an immense curiosity. In four years, the child has accumulated great knowledge. Suddenly the child has an order, a pattern of knowledge. The world opens up.

**About Ruben,
four years old**

After having been a quiet child, our son suddenly became defiant, grumpy, very stubborn and talks incessantly. He is restless and wants activity all the time. It almost drives me nuts. I know he can find things to do on his own.

As the child realizes how big the world is and better understands the threats and dangers, he often becomes more anxious than before. Fears of darkness and nightmares are common. The four-year-old has a good self-esteem and is often pleased with having gotten so big. The child believes in his own ability and enjoys being capable. He looks for adventure further away from mom and dad. But home is still the safe base. The four-year-old loves his family.

The child becomes social

A four-year-old is often willing to cooperate and compromise. However, a four-year-old is not as easy to distract anymore. One can no longer "fool" the child into doing something, like when he was smaller. The four-year-old also wants to understand what is being said and also be the center of attention. If we adults ignore the child, he can get very annoyed.

A four-year-old likes to be big and make decisions and tell his younger siblings how things should be or how they should be done and what little sister may or may not do. It is not certain that these rules apply to the four-year-old himself. He is happy in being a kind of police. The four-year-old needs rules to deal with life and is happy telling them to others. "My dad said that you are not allowed." At this age, the child can, for example, begin to learn traffic rules, but if something exiting happens they may forget them just as fast. Thus, one cannot rely on the child in traffic. Just as one cannot trust that the child will take care of the little brother. Now, the child can really empathize with how other people feel; it can get very involved when someone gets hurt and exclaim, "Poor, poor you."

Friends become increasingly important. They almost become icons for the four-year-old's new and more independent life. And the four-year-old chooses friends on his own. The child can wait for its turn and be considerate in a completely different way than before. Together, children can create rules and organize games. They play at their best if they play two and two, or in small groups. Role-play games are popular and important. Through role-play, they learn to deal with fears and experiences, thoughts and concerns. Many four-year-olds sit in front of the computer and gain new skills and angles of incidence. The four-year-old knows a lot and if he does not, he will find out what he wants to know by asking for an example. There can be a true cross fire of questions. But short answers are enough; they will not listen to long expositions. He is eager and curious and it is fun and rewarding to talk to him. He can often justify his opinion and argue in favor of something. But he is still partly illogical and changes opinions easily. Thought is still magical to a certain point. "If I pat the stone it will probably be happy."

About Hugo, four years old

I am going through a rough period with my four-year-old right now. My son is "always" grumpy, angry and awkward. It makes everything we do boring. If he does not get what he wants, he fights and he kicks. He seeks independence in everything. All the time, he keeps asserting that he is the one in charge and not us. If we tell him to stop doing something he always continues doing it a few more times. He fantasizes a lot and always pretends to be someone else, someone who is older and "better" than him.

I know that a four-year-old has a vivid imagination, but does he not consider himself good enough? Today, for example, he started to play hockey. It went very well and he fought on. Afterwards, he wanted to bring the pads home, and he was not allowed. Then he became furious and started fussing and nagging. In the end I lost my patience because I thought he was being spoiled and ungrateful.

He screamed and screamed. He fussed and nagged. After a long while he calmed down and with a trembling lip he said that he was not a real hockey-guy because they all have protection pads. At night he played that he was a famous hockey player, and of course, best of them all.

Both small and big

There is also a lot going on physically right now. At three years old, the child is still chubby and toddler-like. At four years old, the baby-chubbiness disappears, the child kicks off and the body gets more of an "adult" form. The child becomes increasingly more secure physically. Being able to do the basics such as walking and running is obvious. Now the child practices more difficult things such as balancing or swinging high. It is great to master the body. The instinct of competition appears and the four-year-old competes with both himself and with other children. "Look, now I jumped even higher." Adults should preferably look and admire every time. The joy in mastering the body better and better is great, and sometimes the child goes to the extremes and complicates the movements unnecessarily, adults may think. There is a lot of life in a four-year-old's body; in fact, it is nearly impossible to be still. Though sometimes the child will cuddle up in mom's or in dad's arms, maybe with the thumb in its mouth, and wants to be very small. Four years of age is a time of opposites, just like all transition periods are.

The child also develops a lot intellectually at this age. It can figure out how things work. The child may begin to take interest in letters and numbers. Some put a lot of concentration and attention in letters and some even crack reading codes. Others do not have the patience

**About
Ellen, four and a half years old**

I could hardly believe it was true when I observed how Ellen, together with another two-and-a-half-year-old girl old girl, at the Montessori preschool, took responsibility for the lunch table setting for fifteen children. They ran the table setting all on their own, picked up the correct number of plates, glasses and cutlery and missed nothing, not even the condiments or napkins. At home Ellen is our baby, the little sister she is, and she can barely do anything on her own.

for such things yet. The child is able to tell their whole name and maybe even where it lives.

A four-year-old reflects a lot. What is life, what is death, why do we live, what happened before I existed, and what happens when we die? They both understand and do not understand. She can understand that a bird dies. But the next moment she says, "It will probably start flying again." The child moves freely between understanding and not understanding. Small and big at the same time. One minute the child is big, capable, and arrogant and knows exactly how everything should be. The next minute the child is a toddler in need of a good rest with mom and dad, a child who loves its family. Tough yet sensitive at the same time. One minute he hits his little brother who disturbs his construction. The next moment he hugs him repentantly and lets him borrow his beloved car. Some four-year-olds can handle being away from mom and dad overnight or for a few days. For others it is still too early. Often, we parents know if it would work or not for our own child. Then one can ignore other people's likings on whether it is too early and if the child should do it or not. But of course, if possible it is wise to have a "back-up plan." Be prepared on having to pick up the child who sleeps over for the first time at a friend's house.

About Philip, four years old

We were all sick recently, my wife and I and little sister, our daughter, who is two years old. We had tonsillitis and it was really bad. But Philip was healthy and he withstood it. He felt a responsibility and took care of all of us. He brought us water and tissues, opened the door when someone was there, and answered the phone. He thoughtfully asked if we felt a little better. He was very pleased and proud.

Helpful – at least while away

At daycare it usually works out fine. It is common for four-year-olds to be helpful and efficient; they put on their rain boots, go to the bathroom on their own, and help out with the table setting. But studies

About Olivia, four and a half years old

I am convinced that I am the worst mother in the world, at least to my girl. This past year everything has gotten worse and worse. I am not ashamed about getting angry with her, but I get angry in such a bad way. She screams and cries a lot, she always has. She cries when she wakes up and when she is hungry. She screams because a toy breaks. I fix it and she screams anyways and throws the toy so that it breaks again. She screams because we are out of ice cream or because her little sister got ketchup before her. Sometimes there is nothing more for her to scream over, but she cries anyway. Sometimes I think she wants to scream. She controls a lot in my life and sometimes I get so heartbroken. There are days when I wish she did not exist. Sometimes I snap and tell her the worst things. That she is stupid or that I do not want her. On those occasions I want to hurt her, I want to make her understand that she cannot behave however she wants to. Often I put the blame on her, saying "Look how you are hurting me." I know all of this is wrong, but I can do nothing else. I am supposed to be the steady rock that coped with all kinds of weather.

show there is a difference at daycare between boys and girls. Girls are generally more helpful and "crafty" and remain close to the staff. Boys are tougher and are seen and heard more, at least if the girls are around. But studies and experience show that to a certain extent, it is we adults who contribute to these differences by treating boys and girls differently and that we can change it by changing our adult behavior. The four-year-old is really able to behave if you, for example, go on a visit or to a café. At a child's health center, children are usually very cooperative and find it fun to try to solve tasks and they do it with great seriousness. But it requires a great effort to be big and behave well while away. Therefore, it is not certain that it works just as well at home. At home, the child takes out its tensions and fatigue on the parents and can be whiny and angry. But many parents of four-year-olds talk about how incredibly helpful they are even at home, at least when they feel like it. How the child is supportive if this is needed, how it likes to get responsibility. How it shines with pride when it contributes. Most four-year-olds find it fun to perform practical jobs. They can set the table, help to cook, bake, clean and be a really great help. The child dares to try new things and is able to cooperate.

Mom and Dad are the best

At four years old, gender differences become evident. Many girls love to dress in pink and gold, while boys refuse to wear "girly colors." Children often play differently. The girls stick to the doll corner and the boys construct and build. But children also play a lot across gender boundaries. A four-year-old knows that there is a difference between sexes and is considerate of it. Boys can be sorry that they cannot have children and girls because they do not have penis and cannot stand up and pee.

Family is important for four-year-olds. Mom and dad are the best in the world. Many children at this age are clingy; they do not want to be separated from mom and dad, especially if they are going out on a visit. Then, the tough kid is all of a sudden small and sad. Younger siblings are admittedly difficult, but they are often well-beloved.

65

Furthermore, they are fun – small and ignorant as they are. The four-year-old does not miss an opportunity to talk about how great and talented he is and how childish and small his smaller sibling is. But the love for smaller siblings is sometimes hot and cold. Hugging can suddenly turn into pinching. Sometimes there may be periods of really annoying sibling conflicts. Older siblings and their friends are often idols for the four-year-old. Happy is the four-year-old who is allowed to spend time with big and admired children. When one is in midst of a period of development, changes are rarely welcome. Therefore, it can be difficult to get new siblings. Then, things often turn upside down at home with new routines and a baby who takes up a lot of attention and time. In addition, the big child may perhaps get significantly less time at daycare now, and this can also result in a difficult and big change. But this is often a good time to have a sibling. The four-year-old can understand and accept that a baby takes a lot of mom and dad's time, and many four-year-olds like to cuddle with a baby sibling.

Struggle of the giants

A four-year-old is able to cooperate, but is often everything else but cooperative! The four-year-old can be whiny and refuse and think that everything is wrong. No clothes will do, not that game, not that way home, not now, not later, not this song and so on. And they know exactly how it should be. They think that they know everything and always want to have it their way, even though they often do not even really know what they want.

In such situations, as a parent it is important to oppose. Then the four-year-old argues back and learns that a good argument often wins, and this becomes a good lesson. But the child should not always win. It requires resistance. Life with a four-year-old can often be described as the struggle of the giants with violent clashes, a struggle is which all resources are allowed. Earlier, life with the child had been quite simple and close. Sometime around the age of four, you enter into a dead end and feel totally helpless. The strategies used in the past for the

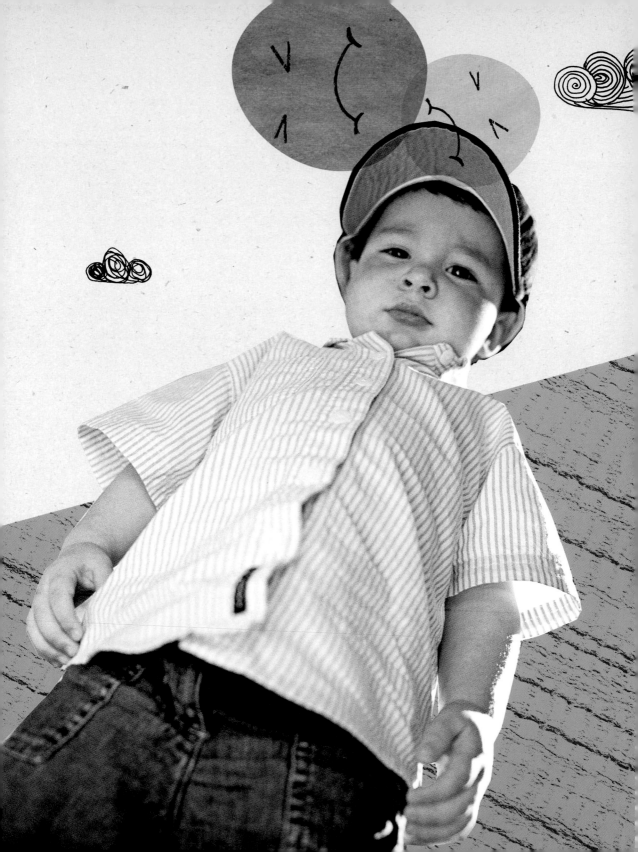

About Noah, just over four years old

He is so incredibly positive to everything. When we go on an outing he pours praise on everything and on everyone. What a nice house, the good food, how lucky we are with the weather, what fun we have, how lucky we are after all, how fun it is to be on an outing. But when we are going on a visit somewhere the fights never end. It seems that he is not able to break up. After half an hour of battle I start shouting or crying. Then he slowly gives up his battle. It is almost as is if he needs all that fighting.

upbringing and socializing with the child no longer work. There can be a chaos at home. While away on a visit, the child is often nice to deal with and mom and dad are praised for their child. But they themselves feel totally unsuccessful.

They hear themselves say and do things they never thought about themselves. But this entire struggle is necessary! In all their strength and sensitivity, children actually need struggles. Now as a parent, we must teach how life is outside of the family, how to be a more mature person – more adult with all that this entails. They are no longer toddlers and one day they will leave us to fend for themselves. And life is not always easy and friendly.

You can no longer whine and scream and believe that everyone else will understand and do as you please. Many of us parents who imagined a democratic and "tranquil" upbringing where we would correct our child with calm, become quite distraught when we are not able to remain calm and instead start yelling and screaming, and maybe even grabbing the child violently. We think we failed completely and accuse ourselves. I, the parent of the child who loves her most of all, am the one who gets so mad at her and behaves so wrongly.

This battle is so hard, sometimes you feel as if you do not like the kid. But it is the job of parents to battle with the child and help her out of this confused state that the four years of age implies. But despite all the fights, screams, and threats, the child trusts in the fact that it is loved by mom and dad and they help it to mature and develop. Thus, the child needs our anger and our resistance. One is not only allowed to get terribly angry with one's errant four-year-old, but one should and needs to get angry.

Fears

Since the four-year-old knows and is able to do so much, the world can be daunting. The child realizes that there is a lot it cannot understand and control and this is scary. He has begun to realize how big the world is and this can be frightening. The four-year-old does not dare to see scary things on TV anymore. Fear of darkness is common. We parents may experience all of this as nonsense and wimpiness. A year ago, when the child was younger, it dared to go into a dark room, and then there was no talk of monsters and villains. But the four-year-old's fear of ghosts, monsters, and darkness is not wimpiness and it does not necessarily mean that the child is insecure. It is all about imagination and development. What may hide in the dark? What if there are ghosts!

The greater the child's ability is to fantasize about life and everything that is going on, the greater are the fears. But the child is also increasing its capacity to tackle fear and eventually moves on with life, stronger and more mature.

About Tuva, four years old

Sometimes Tuva and I get so terribly angry at each other and we scream and fuss and fight. The other day, after we both had calmed down, I asked her how she felt when we were fighting. Then she answered "I feel in my heart that I need to fight with you." It was so nice to hear, because, of course, I have such a guilty conscience about screaming and arguing.

About Lisa, four years old

Oftentimes I have such a guilty conscience because I cannot stand my little Lisa. She can drive me completely mad and I become exactly the mother I do not want to be. Immature, inconsistent, and wrong in every way. I feel ashamed of myself, but I just cannot handle the situation. My partner (who is not the father of the child) has much more patience with her. But she is not as bad with him either. I have also felt as a failure, that he can handle her better than I can, though he is not even her father. But when I talked about it with a friend who is a child psychologist she said that I should take it as a compliment that the girl is harder on me. She says it is because she and I are so close, so she kind of dares to be defiant and troublesome with me.

Fear will pass faster if we carefully guide the child through it. Allow the child to crawl into the parental bed, turn on the light in the bedroom and receive the child with warmth. It is also common that the child has nightmares and gets night terrors.

A good way to overcome fear is to play. Many children in this age pretend that they are Batman, Superman, or Spiderman. Then the child can subdue to fear, handle it, and take power over it. The four-year-old has a great deal of imagination and often lives in a fairytale world where there might be people and animals only they know about. Imaginary friends are common. Four-year-olds often have a quite casual way of dealing with the truth, adults may think. However, children at this age have a hard time distinguishing between fantasy and reality, truth and untruth. Therefore, things go wrong when we accuse the child of lying. For the child, this imagination is real. It is only later on that the child learns to distinguish between fantasy and reality. A child who "lies" a lot at this age has an abundant imagination.

THINGS TO CONSIDER

→ Children have many questions and concerns, and they need answers for them.

→ The four-year-old is both small and dependent, and big and capable.

→ The child needs the right amount of rules to stick to.

→ Let your child be involved in baking, cooking, cleaning and more.

→ Let the child take the right amount of responsibility.

→ Struggle and resistance is needed.

→ Take the child's fears seriously.

→ Your child may be an angel while away and horrible at home. This is just as it should be.

→ Let friends, both real and imaginary, take place in the child's life. They are important!

→ A four-year-old who "lies" has a very abundant imagination.

→ Four-year-olds are wise and constructive. Ask your child for help if you do not know what to do in different situations, such as in hassles around food and sleep.

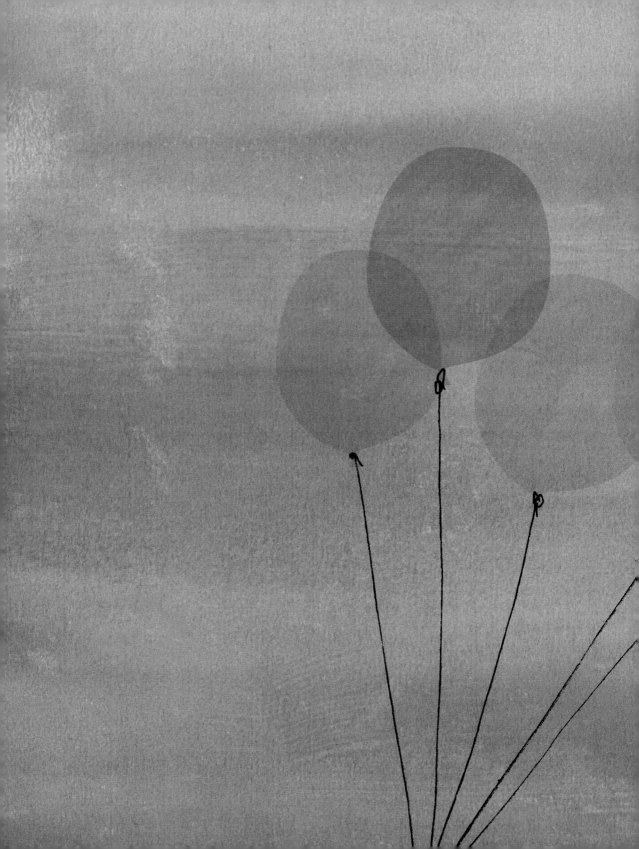

Six years old — little teenage years

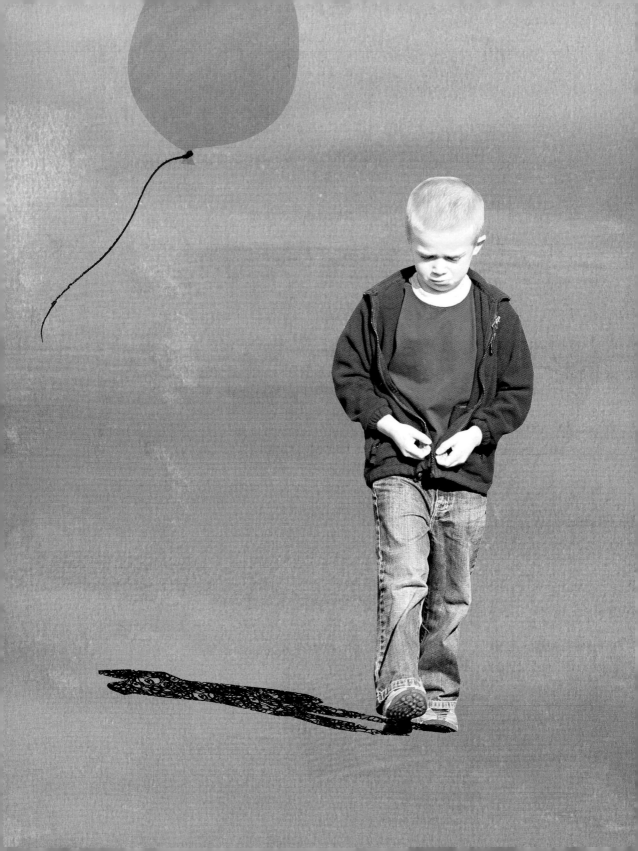

A SIX-YEAR-OLD IS about to become big and kicks off in both body and soul. Arms and legs grow, the proportions of the body become more like an adult, and the child has anxiety in the body. The spiritual development is at least as big and exiting. There is an ongoing struggle for liberation, a struggle between being independent and dependent, between being small and big. The child is usually both sensitive and easily wounded and often finds it difficult to take criticism.

This development is similar to the one occurring in adolescence, and age six is therefore usually referred to as the little teens. It can be a messy period with all these concerns, both for the child and for the parents. But it passes! The six-year-old is very eager to learn and wants proper answers. As an adult you can easily become stumped when confronted by a six-year-old who asks challenging follow-up questions if you try to get away with a simple answer. At six years, the child gets something which can be called an outlook on life. She has a concept of time and learns the clock. She is stubborn and knows what she wants. But the child is also good at compromising and understands consequences in an entirely different way than before.

She can take arguments and argue cleverly on her own, because now she masters language. The child does not buy your arguments offhand, but rather contradicts them.

75

The six-year-old thinks very clearly and logically, and is a fast learner. Now, many become seriously interested in letters and numbers, if they have not already learned them before. A lot is going on. They lose teeth and learn to swim. Fairness is important and it can be tedious to create fairness between siblings now. "Why does she get it and not me?" is a common reply. It must all be fair and square.

Moderate responsibility

You can usually rely on a six-year-old and he likes to get tasks and responsibility. He can for example take responsibility for younger siblings in a completely different way than before. But there is of course a difference between different children. Some take responsibility better than others. A child can go to the store and buy something on its own or take the bus to town and be met by somebody there. Another six-year-old would be able to run across the street or get off the bus at the wrong place, while a third child would become anxious and frightened by all this responsibility.

About Marus, six years old

His thirst for knowledge is immense. How tall can the palms grow? How high can the waves get? By the way, how many waves are there at the same time? How can you know if this gold is real? Thousands upon thousands of questions and he has learned how to figure things out on his own. He searches in books and checks online, and asks and asks.

There are no rules for how much responsibility you can put on a six-year-old. It is of course the parents who know their own children and are able to give responsibility on a moderate level. To be given moderate responsibility reinforces the child's self-esteem and helps it develop and mature. The child grows, partly due to the parents giving it responsibility and partly by coping with the task. At six years, children feel very confident with their parents. The child relies on the parents' love, and both mom and dad are important. Getting along with siblings at this age is usually no problem. However, it can be troublesome to have younger siblings who destroy each other's stuff and interfere in important tasks. On other occasions the six-year-old plays with his younger siblings and other small children. A six-year-old can take initiatives and organize games, keep track of the smaller kids and be admired by them. And praise is something that the six-year-old cannot get enough of.

At this time, the child takes a big step into social life. They are able to create their own relationship with a friend or with the teacher at school. But friends are of course the most important. It is important to be accepted and to blend in. The child wants to be "like everyone else," have the same clothes, the same hairstyle and the same rules. The child wants to assert himself and starts to compare himself with others and see himself through the eyes of others. Children compete in everything: how many teeth they have lost, how many Lego pieces they have, and so on. It seems like a neverending story.

Now it is often exiting to spend the night at grandma's or a friend's house, even though if at bedtime one can become small and want to come home. But the six-year-old can take arguments. If she cannot be picked up, she accepts it and is able to sleep away even though she longs for home.

About Betty, age six and a half

Her spiteful period began when she was two to three years old and has persisted until recently. Initially, she was violently angry. At age six, she was sulky and bitter. She was unresponsive and quiet when she was upset. She had a tough time, but then, at school, she made new friends. Now everything is much more calm. It's not just adults who have a life outside of the home that affects how we feel.

Fun and friends

At this age, there is often a big difference between girls' and boys' games and drawings. Boys play war, and girls dress up as lovely ladies and ballet dancers. They draw princesses, flowers, and houses. There are certainly innate differences, but there are studies that have shown

Sometimes it is okay to be angry and sometimes not. Sometimes I get so angry that I almost get a little sad. Then I go to a place where I can be left alone. I someone comes I tell them to go away. But sometimes I wish that they would not care about me telling them to "go away." Then, I want them to stay, but I do not say it.

how we adults affect children so that these differences become too big, both in terms of games and behavior. We push children into patterns and limit them, we encourage boys for example to help themselves and to take up space, and girls to show empathy and to express themselves with words. By changing our behavior, we can give children the freedom to develop different sides. In the book *Girls, Boys and Pedagogues* by Kajsa Wahlstrom you can read more. Boys and girls often play separately, but also in large, big, and mixed groups. Mainly girls have best friends who often change from day to day, or week to week, but they also play in groups. If more than two children play it can happen that they are mean to each other. "You are not allowed to be with us" and similar things can be heard. Children often play semi-secret games. For example, they can close themselves in and play doctor. They know a whole lot about sex and "banned" words, and these concepts very exciting to explore. There can be a lot of giggling about sex, and there are competitions regarding who is the most daring.

Many spend frequent and long hours in front of the computer, both alone and with other children. Computer games play an important role for the six-year-old who can exercise both coordination and the ability to react, while gaining knowledge and additional excitement and entertainment. Now the child can even handle board games. They quickly learn the rules and follow them. But six-year-olds tend to be bad losers and condone the adults who sometimes let them win.

Time of changes

There is a lot happening around the child when it is six years old. The biggest change is that they start preschool. Daycare is over and

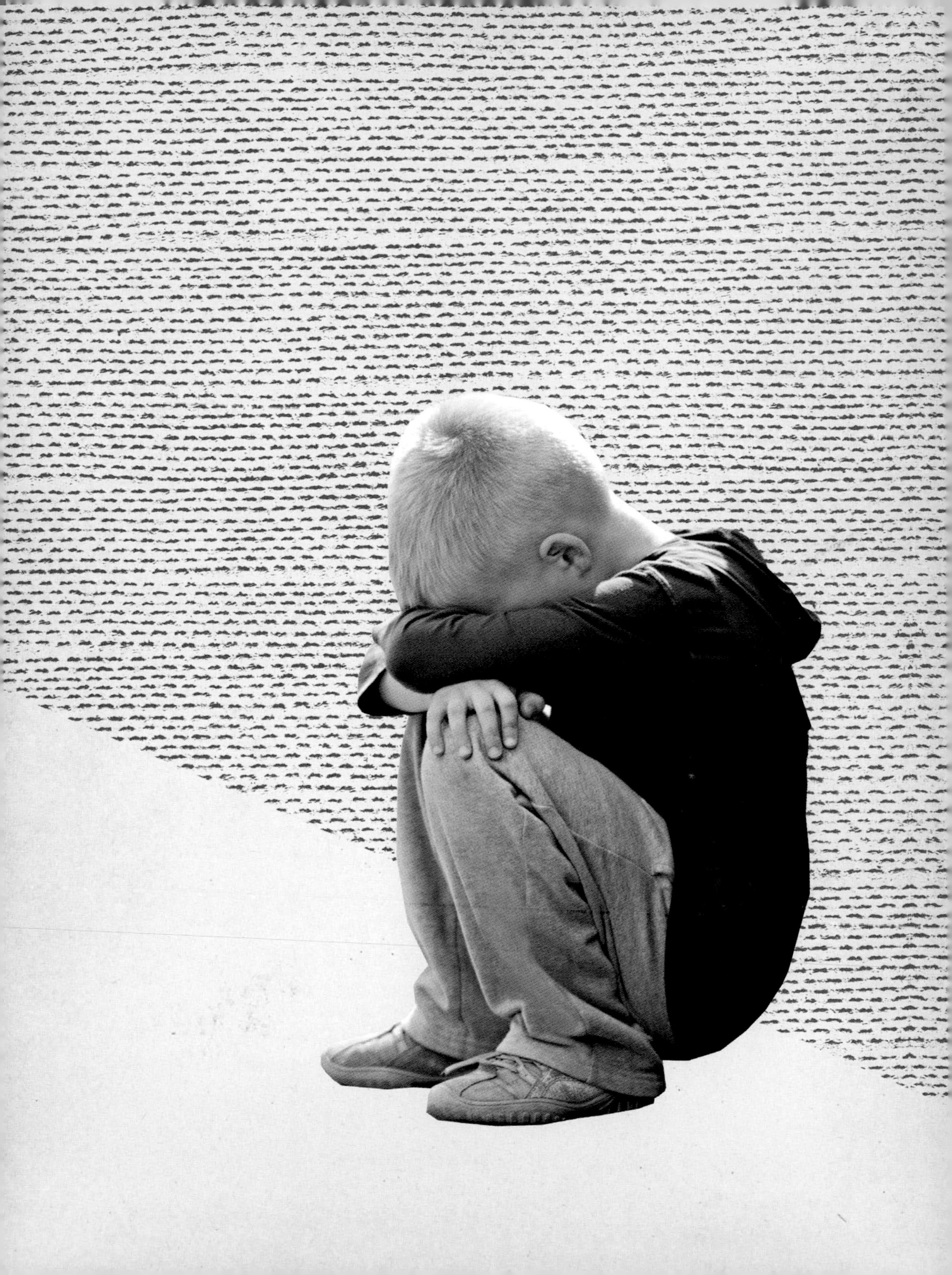

About Alice, just over
six years old

It is tough to say goodbye. She likes to be at daycare but there are such ceremonies each day when we part. She follows me through the daycare courtyard waving and saying all the goodbye words she can think of, and I have to wave and answer her each time. Hugging and kissing rituals must be exactly the same every morning otherwise it will all go wrong.

now the child is supposed to function in a bigger group and in a different way than before, leaving a safe place with familiar routines and having to fulfill new demands. They are required to sit still and they should be able to follow instructions in a different way than before. Leaving the old for the new and unknown can feel exiting and like an "at last" for a child who is tired of daycare and who looks forward to greater challenges. For another child, it can feel awful and sad to leave the security of the daycare world and be forced into the new and unknown. But most six-year-olds can handle changes pretty well after a while, even difficult things like moving or parents divorcing. The child may cry and long, but most can handle the situation after a period of sadness and anger.

Thoughts of death often occupy the six-year-old. He knows what death means. The child also knows that it can partially fend for himself. Meanwhile, he is fully aware that he is still small and totally dependent on mom and dad. The child realizes that one day it will have to do without mom and dad, and this can create severe anxiety. At this age there are often protracted farewell ceremonies and even tucking in at night can be protracted. This is all related to the child's new insights. The child knows what a good bye can mean – it may actually be that you will never see each other again. Death lurks around the corner. Such feelings are natural and not harmful and form part of maturation. However, the child may feel the need to talk about death. There can be nice and close talks with the six-year-old if and when he wants. It is common for the child to dream a lot during this time, and often these are horrible dreams about death and murder and about being chased. Then it might be nice and important to have access to mom and dad's bed again and be small.

Anxiety in the body

The six-year-old cannot sit still. He flies around and is not still for even one minute. He sways high, very high, the next second he is in front of the computer and then throws himself right into an exciting fantasy-game. Happy, restless, and like a cat on hot bricks. The whole time she wants to show off, get praise and get attention: look at me diving or biking, balancing on the railing and swaying the highest of all.

A six-year-old can hang upside down from the couch armrest and watch television. The child twists and turns, rocks the chair, semi-sitting and semi-laying, posturing and prancing. A pediatrician who has met thousands of six-year-olds before they start school told me that hardly any of them are able to sit still on the chair for that little moment they spend at the doctor without sooner or later falling off of the chair. There are theories about this bodily anxiety and one of them is that the skeleton is growing rapidly at six years of age. Surrounding tendons and muscles grow slower and cannot really keep up. Therefore, the child bends and elongates its legs, performs all kinds of stretch movements and fidgets. Psychosomatic symptoms are very common, especially stomachaches. It is estimated that approximately one-third of all six-year-olds have such symptoms.

There tends to be a lot of nagging about sitting properly and not running around. But the six-year-old can often not hold back the turmoil in his body; he has no control over it. Another troublesome situation, especially for the children themselves, is that their precision and coordination skills are now worse than before. The child tends to get careless, clumsy, and awkward, and is not able to control his body like before. The child, who previously was able pour juice from a pitcher without any problems, now pours it on the side or tips the glass

81

**About Lovisa,
age six**

I am really afraid that mom and dad will die and I cry every night, but mom and dad do not know about it. I think that if I tell them something may happen to them.

over with the pitcher. As a parent you can get both surprised and angry. One knows that the child has in fact been able to pour nicely for several years. Why is it so careless and unconcentrated now? It might be nice for both parents and children to know that there are physical causes. The six-year-old is very aware of his failure and wants to be big and skilled. But in order to mask those feelings he often messes up a little bit more and makes a big deal out of his clumsiness. He may play a buffoon and for example, pour sloppily.

However, at age six, children may pull themselves together and in certain situations they can be calm and focused. This makes us even more annoyed; we know that the child is able. There is usually a lot of nagging and fighting. "Sit still at the dinner table," or "Watch it! I know you can," and the like. At best, the child makes an attempt to "behave" but soon it is impossible again.

Anxiety in the soul

Six-year-olds test limits, they push limits and verify what is allowed and what is not. Telling wild stories and bragging form part of boundary testing. The fact that the six-year-old doesn't always stick completely to the truth does not need to be taken into account very seriously. The six-year-old really believes in himself and at the same time, he has huge doubts about his own abilities. Doubts occupy the child very much and he is often self-critical. "Who am I?, Ugh, I'm so ugly. I can't do anything." The child has high demands on himself, and needs a lot of support, appreciation, and praise.

Six-year-olds seek their identity, they play superheroes or princesses as a way to test themselves. Big and small, cowardly and brave, happy and sad, independent and dependent, pessimistic and optimistic. It can change fast. Behind the tough facade is a sensitive soul. The six-year-old is fragile, and self-esteem is slightly chipped at its edges.

Six-year-olds can get stomachaches from worries and anxiety, but also in anticipation of something fun. It is common that among friends the child is tough and loud, sure of himself, and knows and is able to do everything. At home, he can show his "little" sides, ask for help, curl up in your lap and hug, and be pampered and cry out.

Obsessions are common and a way to rule the world, to get a handle on it. The child wants, for example, to do the same thing many times, or do things in a specific order, otherwise it will be completely wrong. They can get ideas like that there is a kind of film on the LEGO pieces that needs to be rubbed off. Magical thinking is close to obsessions and is also common at age six. The child may be terrified that something will happen, but does not dare to tell anyone about these feelings because then the fears may come true. Or, the child thinks that if the next car is green, something bad will happen and if it is red something good will happen.

> **About Emil, almost 6 years**
>
> He is so complicated! If he gets his shoes on when we are about to go to daycare, they need to fit perfectly, and me and his little sister must go out the door exactly when he says so, otherwise he needs to take his shoes off and start over. Sometimes he changes his mind on the way and then we have to start all over again, otherwise he becomes hysterical. And although he just peed before we left, he must stop on the way to daycare to pee. Daycare is two minutes away. If he has a cold he must blow his nose again and again even though nothing comes out, because it feels "so weird." I get very annoyed with all this hassle, especially when I am tired. Unfortunately, I cannot help but show my annoyance.

The child needs resistance

All of this that goes on in a six-year-old's body and mind makes many six-year-olds considerably unruly. The child can become fussy, irritable,

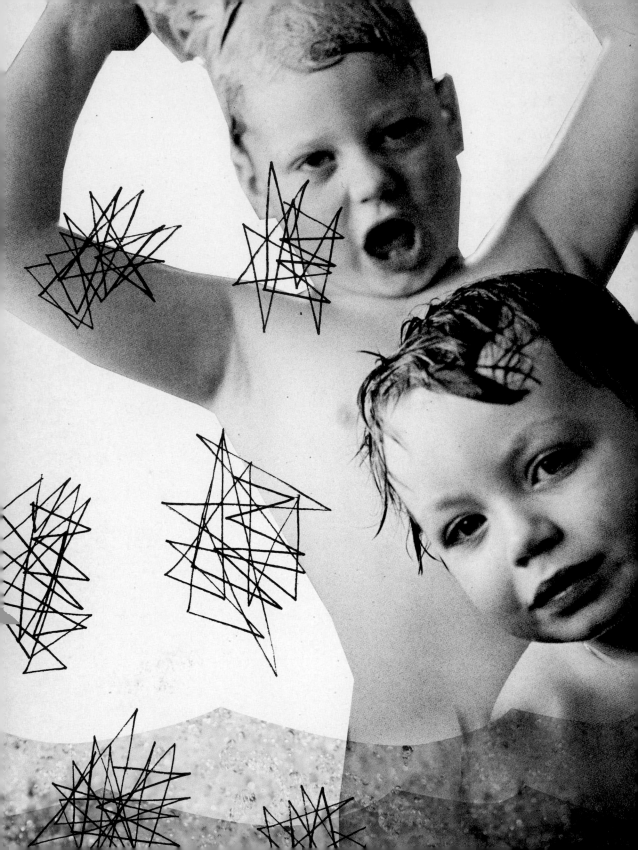

and angry. Nothing is good enough, the child can suffer something close to melancholy. But since this is the period of opposites, these blues will soon turn into joy of life.

It is important to remember that this image of six-year-olds is not true for everyone. Many are in a peaceful and harmonious state at six. Instead, they became unruly earlier and have already gotten out of their "six-year-old-defiance," or they enter it later. Others are never really bothersome. But many have severe temper tantrums at age six, outbursts similar to those at age two to three. They can throw themselves on the floor and scream.

There are six-year-olds who already worked their way through an angry and aggressive period and now they turn moody and sad instead and take a step back in conflicts. They have learned to handle their emotions in a more adult way now. Now, we parents have even less patience than when the child was younger since we know that the child has much more understanding. We do not expect a two-year-old to understand and obey, but we do expect it from a six-year-old. Therefore, we also become much angrier at the six-year-old.

When we have fought long and without any success, the only thing that remains is screaming and yelling. But most parents do not want to get so angry at their children to the extent of feeling guilty. But we are not bad parents if we yell and scream. The situation and the child

Erik, father of boys who are six and three years old

I love my children, and every morning I wake up with good intentions: Today I will be a good and mature parent. But too often I fall asleep sorry and ashamed over failing again. Above all, my youngest son provokes me tremendously and then I can become like a child myself. I stand and roar like a three-year-old or blame the kids by feeling sorry for myself. Or I punish them in a childish and immature way. Some days I am really not proud of myself as a father. I met some friends a few weeks ago and we got to talk about children and parenting. I told them about how hard I find it to be sometimes, and then it turned out that the others felt or had felt in a very similar way. It was actually a great relief to hear that.

85

About Ulli, six and a half years old

Ulli played with her friend Vera for hours without interruption and with great passion. Then she said giggling: "Imagine what one could create out of a little bit of reality and fantasy. We pretended that the mattress was a red dress!"

require this resistance. That does not mean that we do not love our child. The child knows it, even though it might say, "You do not love me."

It is not always easy to get along with a six-year-old and know how to behave towards her. But it is certainly more difficult to be six years old. To come to the edge so often, or to be at odds with the people the child loves the most – us parents – is difficult. The child may also feel guilt and be sad when clashes arise. But this is how it has to be. This is development. Six-year-olds are often wise and constructive.

Therefore, it may be a good solution to ask the child for help if you get stuck in a conflict or a problem. Tell the child that you do not know what to do and ask, "What do you think that we should do?" For example, if the child is difficult to wake up in the mornings, you can ask what to do about it, and the child may suggest their own alarm clock or a mobile wake-up call, or some kind of a reward.

THINGS TO CONSIDER

→ Children need adults who explain the rules clearly.

→ Explain to the child why they may feel anxious in their body.

→ Give the child resistance.

→ Let your child sleep in or near your bed if she is anxious and restless. Do not make a big deal out of it, but just quietly arrange it to make it work.

→ Be tactful. Do not tell others what you think your child would not want to reveal, for example, that the child is sleeping in your bed, that they wet the bed or do not dare to sleep alone. And hold back on "baby-cuddling" when friends are looking.

→ Give the child the right amount of responsibility.

→ Let your child be small when they need it.

→ Make sure that life is not too structured with various activities, so that there is time to "do nothing" and play freely.

→ Let your child find their way to a sport or leisure activity that fits. And let the activity be pleasurable and play-oriented, not competition-oriented.

→ Take the child's worries, such as about death, seriously. Do not dismiss with "I will not die" or similar. Say instead "If I could decide, I would never die or be away from you" or something similar.

→ Accept if the child makes things up, but put a stop to it if the lies affect others.

→ Do not force yourself on your six-year-old with hugs and kisses, but rather wait for the child to come to you when it wants to cuddle.

→ If you are concerned that the child has many obsessions, or if you feel worried for some other reason and your concern persists, you can contact a private child psychologist.

→ If you and the child are in a "fighting" period, it can be nice and liberating to sometimes, when the situation is calm, talk to the child about how it feels for the child and for yourself.

→ Let your child help if you are stuck on a problem.

USEFUL READING

The books about Mardie by Astrid Lindgren.
The books about Pippi Longstocking by Astrid Lindgren.
The books about Alfie Atkins by Gunillam Bergström.
The books about Zackarina and the sand wolf by Åsa Lind.
Brenda Brave by Astrid Lindgren.
Lotta on Troublemaker Street by Astrid Lindgren.

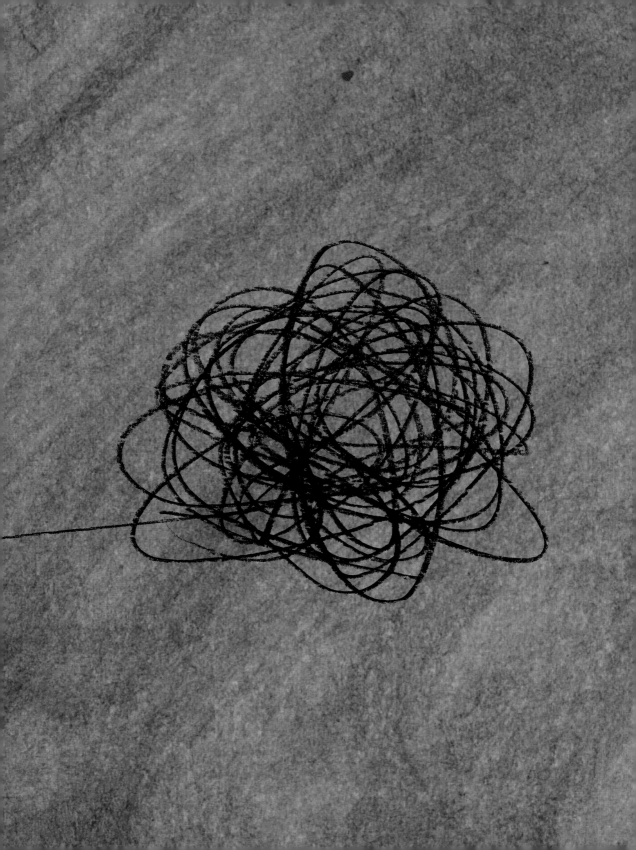

Extra-demanding children — more of everything

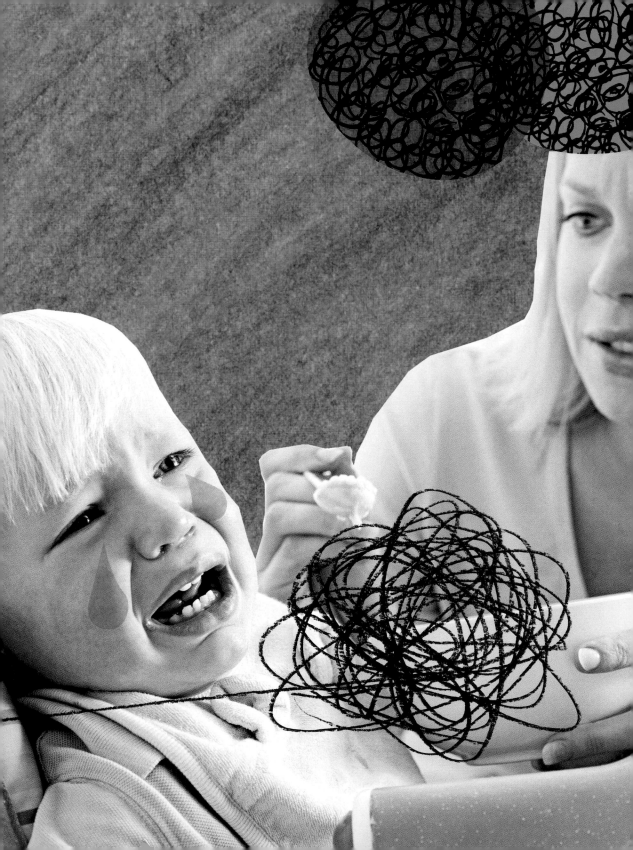

⇶ EXTRA-DEMANDING CHILDREN – MORE OF EVERYTHING

SOME CHILDREN are extraordinarily demanding. They are also unusually full of life and vigor. They are stubborn, intense and strong-willed about their preferences, and they are often early in their development, and intelligent and sensitive. These children's senses are well developed and they often experience more than others. They hear, see, feel, taste and smell exceptionally well. Therefore, they easily become overloaded by impressions, especially in environments where there is a lot going on and after intensive days. This can result in severe outbursts.

Their emotional expressions are strong. When they get angry or grumpy they become *extremely* angry or grumpy. When they are happy they are often very happy and pleased. In short: they have and they are more of everything. One can describe these children as diamonds that have to be sanded in order to then become jewels. They have a strength and fantasy to envy them for and which will take them far in their lives. Sometimes we call them the four-percent-children, since about four children out of one hundred are such children.

When the strong child is in the midst of a period of defiance and resistance, it is easy to believe that it will always be like that. But then the difficulties suddenly fade away and the child enters a calmer phase and does not have as strong outbursts. The child rests before it enters a new difficult period. When these kinds of children enter an obstinate age, it is of course more exhausting to be a parent.

Controlling parents and siblings

The more stubborn a child is, the more it fights to resist. These unusually strong children can control the whole family with an iron fist. They can even rock the relationship between mom and dad. They have great power. The extra-stubborn children constantly challenge their parents and their patience. Therefore, it is difficult being their parent. During some periods, they can actually create a total chaos and despair and completely dominate the life of the rest of the family.

It may be difficult for others to understand how these children are. Often, they are easy to deal with when they are at daycare, school, or away on a visit. It is up to us parents to encourage the children to show their true defiant, angry, or whiny sides with the assurance of being loved anyway.

The unusually demanding children think more than other children. Their brain is booming. They think about what will happen in advance, and since they have a great imagination they imagine how things will be. Then, if things do not turn out as they had imagined, they can have a real breakdown. There can be a kind of explosion and the child goes insane. It can scream, "I am useless, I am stupid" or something similar. As parents, we interpret it as the child having poor self-esteem.

But it is not about that. It is rather the opposite. It is an expression of their confusion. These children often have a high sense of self-esteem but not precisely in these kinds of difficult situations or during certain periods. The unusually stubborn children make us feel like failed parents because we have to be

**About Jonas,
nineteen months old**

My son whines so much that it drives me completely crazy. Nothing is right, nothing is good enough, least of all me. Sitting in the stroller is wrong, pushing the stroller on his own is wrong, being carried is wrong. Eating on his own is wrong, but being fed is also wrong. This is how I feel in my despair, at least on some days. He rules my life completely. The worst part is that he is still not satisfied. Sometimes it is difficult to like him.

92

close to them, yell at them, exhort and tell them what they can and cannot do.

As a parent one tends to take on the blame; we think we have been too tolerant or too strict, too demanding or too angry, or too inconsistent. We think that we have failed to set limits. But it is not the parents' fault that the child is unusually stubborn or strong. Some children are like this. They need to have their strong outbursts in order to bring order to their inner world which is full of thoughts, feelings, and events. There is nothing wrong with this, nothing negative. But it is really difficult and tiring.

An extra-powerful child requires and obviously needs extra strong resistance. Therefore, there are strong reactions from both children and parents with such a child at home. These reactions are followed by crying, closeness and reconciliation.

About Valerie, three years old

My daughter has always had a quick temper and a strong will ever since she was very little. She is a bit too "thick skinned." She defies and defies, whines, and does everything just the opposite way. She refuses to eat at every meal. She whines and I raise my voice and shout. I feel very guilty afterwards. But I think that I will certainly not give in, and I am sure she thinks the same thing.

What can we do?

The usual parenting methods are not really made for these extra-stubborn children, other regulations need to be applied. One cannot be as consistent with them as with other children, but one has to give in more. Children know the rules and what is right, but they refuse to abide. Therefore, one has to let the children decide more, otherwise there will be too much fighting.

The fact that the four-percent-children are unusually creative and imaginative is something we parents can utilize. We can try to find unusual, imaginative solutions when things become difficult, solutions that suit our own child. Making exceptions and not being consistent fit the extra demanding children, or as Oscar Wilde put it, "Consistency is the last refuge for those who lack imagination."

About Charlotte, one and a half years old

Our daughter is lively, loud, and strong-willed. And that is just fine. But our entire existence is tested every day. What should you do when you have such a wild child?

We need to talk to the extra stubborn children as if they were "adults." We can and should include them in our reasoning in a different way than we usually do with children in their age. They can provide startling, wise, and constructive answers because they are intelligent and imaginative.

For example, if we have had an unusually difficult situation with the child the day before, we can ask: "If we could have started over, what should I have done so that it would have been better?" We might also ask: "What should I do next time this happens?"

Since children have extra sensitive and well-developed senses, they can become "overloaded" in busy environments where there is a lot going on and then they can easily have outbursts of anger. Therefore, it may be good to talk to the child before going to an amusement park or to some noisy event. Together with the child we can find solutions and strategies such as walking away now and then. These children need to pause more than others. It can be a good idea to sometimes completely avoid taking these extra-demanding children to the mall on Saturdays and similar.

The child can also get overwhelmed by impressions at daycare as well as at school if there is a lot going on around them, and for example, during games and sports. Since the child does not have their outbursts while away but only when they come home, it is good to talk to teachers and leaders and explain that the child must be allowed to take things at their own pace. Maybe the child needs to sit down and just watch or withdraw for a moment.

Write down the rules

Clear rules at home about things that usually create battles are important for these children. It is helpful to write down the rules, and feel free to put them up on the wall. When battles arise we can point out the rules or read them to the child. It is also important to be clear in our expressions, and say "Come and eat!" instead of saying "Can you come and eat now?" Say "Now it is bedtime!" and not "Is it not time for you to go to bed now?"

Avoid saying "Not." Say, "Now we will clean your room!" rather than "Why do we not clean your room now?" Say "Let's go home!" and not "Should we not go home now?" Children need this help. It is often a good idea to grab the child and look straight in the eye when you lay down the rules. And it is better to say a definite "Stop!" than just saying "No." It becomes clearer and these children need clarity.

About Kalle, three and a half years old

I know that we are not supposed to force children, not yell at them, and always be firm but still kind. But after three and a half years with Kalle, I am exhausted and cannot do it, I yell and nag. I feel sorry about the effect that this will have on him. The worst things is that right there and then, I do not like him. And I definitely do not like the father that I have become.

They also need to be prepared for dinner or bedtime or for school-time. They find it difficult to interrupt what they are doing. It is therefore good to forewarn a moment before. It might be a good idea to give the child an egg timer – when it sounds, it is time. Children are dependent on fixed routines and can become anxious when, for various reasons, the routines change. In such situations, it is also important to forewarn and prepare the child. It is also important to reaffirm the child. When they have an outburst or react strongly in any other way, we tell the child that we see that. We can for example say, "Now you are sad and angry. I understand that, but . . ." So we are not supposed to say, "This is nothing to get angry over."

About Gustav, two years old

To be honest, it is us parents who live at Gustav's place. He is the one who makes the decisions at home.

The four-percent-children often find their own special interests in which they become very talented. This is something good and positive and we should encourage it. Extra-demanding children often have a good sense of humor. So it is good if we parents try to

95

About Jon, three years old

At daycare he is a cinch, the staff tells us. Likewise, he is very manageable when he is with grandpa and grandma. Of course, this feels good in many ways. It would be worse if everyone complained about him. At the same time, I am so tired of hearing everyone say how kind Jon is. If only they knew! They must think I am a strange and unnatural mother who thinks this good child is so difficult.

address them with humor. But it is of course not always easy when the battle is raging and you cannot cope with the situation. Since these children are smart, they are often good at compromising and negotiating. They know it can be a good way to negotiate what they want. This is of course something we parents can take advantage of. We can suggest compromises and negotiations to the children.

As said, these extra lively children are rarely mentally immature. But they are very childish. For example, it is not uncommon for them to want to use diapers when they poop up to age four or five. And since we parents know that they know how to poop on the potty or toilet, there is often a lot of struggle around it. But this battle needs to be discontinued because it is completely meaningless. But it might be good to ask the child when it thinks it will stop pooping in the diaper. They will many times say "When I am five years old" or "When I start school." Why children want to poop in the diaper is something we do not know. Perhaps it's because the unusually well-developed children need to have a childish trait left or they need something they can decide for themselves.

Alphabet kids are something else

Concerns about the so-called medical diagnoses, for example ADHD, have increased in recent years. Many parents of extra demanding children wonder if their child might be a so-called literal child or have serious concentration problems. But children who are "nice while away and difficult at home" do not have any disturbances. But if the child is always very difficult, and the idea that there might be something wrong remains, one can contact a private psychologist for advice and support.

About Anton, two years old

Our son gets so incredibly angry, I cannot even count how many times a day it happens. When he is not screaming, he is very happy, playful, caring, funny, and intelligent. I am proud of him and love him very much. But sometimes I could throw him out the window or jump out myself instead. It starts when he wakes up. He lies in my bed screaming, whining, and being grumpy. This goes on and on throughout the whole day. He gets mad because something does not work as he would like it to, because he is bored, because of everything possible and impossible. He wakes up screaming three to six times during the night.

Sometimes he calms down when I get angry, or if threaten to close the door or something similar. We have a baby too, so we do not get a lot of sleep. I know we should not take it so seriously and that it will pass, but all of this wisdom is not really helping us right now. I get stomachache every now and then and my husband is starting to get stomach problems too. We feel that Anton is breaking us down.

I tend to be calm, but Anton makes me lose my patience. I know it does not help me but I cannot help myself, I get so furious. I not only see red, I see orange sometimes. The worst part is that he is always screaming. Sometimes it feels like I cannot breathe. My husband and I very rarely fight, but when our boy has his tear-away-days, it cannot be avoided.

THINGS TO CONSIDER

→ The unusually demanding children are often precocious, talented, imaginative, and sensitive.

→ They need unusually strong opposition from their parents and can handle it without getting inhibited.

→ Their emotions are unusually strong. They are both angrier and happier than other children.

→ They are sensitive to noisy environments because they pick up on so many impressions. Then they have to walk away or take a break.

→ One cannot be as consistent with them but one has to give in more. Otherwise there will be too much fighting.

→ They are imaginative and it is good to work with imaginative solutions that suit the child.

→ Clear rules are a help, and even better if written down.

→ They need to be prepared and forewarned when something is about to be changed.

→ They need clear reprimands such as "Now it is bedtime."

→ They are good at negotiating and compromising. Take advantage of it.

→ They need confirmation of their feelings, such as, "Now you are really angry."

→ They often have a good sense of humor. Respond to them with humor whenever you can.

→ They often have a special interest. Encourage it.

→ When it is at its hardest to be a parent, try to remember what you have is a diamond, even though it is in its rough state!

USEFUL READING

Raising your Spirited Child by Mary Sheedy Kurcinka.

About Isak, five years old:
"I try everything but nothing works"

When Isak was born, his brother Samuel was three years old and he was a very determined child. Little did we know about what was coming. Little brother Isak somehow plays in an entirely different league. We noticed early on that he had a temper and an iron will. And then it became more and more noticeable. He was the worst at about age three. Then he got terrible outbursts of anger several times a day. But only at home, parents, and to some extent towards his older brother, who is now eight years old. At daycare and with family and friends he is still kind, calm, and charming, a real ray of sunshine. When something goes against his will, he screams. When we lived in an apartment it all went so far that a neighbor made a complaint about us, saying that it was always so loud at our place.

For a while we tried earplugs in order to be able to take it. We have also become used to becoming a bit of a spectacle; people on the street or on the bus stare and probably think what a failure as parents we are.

A few years ago when he was at his worst, on an ordinary morning he would lie down on the floor and just roar. After I helped him get dressed and then went to his older brother to help him with something, Isak would tear off the clothes he had just put on for daycare. Many times it ended with his older brother having to stand and wait in the hallway. It was hopeless and every morning when I got to work, I was exhausted. My job was almost like vacation for a while.

Over the past year, he has learned to deal a little better with his anger and his strong will, and sometimes he participates in finding solutions to the conflicts. But he can still be a force of nature. For example, he will still tear off his jacket outside in freezing cold weather just because his sweater is not on "right." Or refuse to open his mouth when we are about to brush his teeth, refuse to go to the bathroom before going to bed and other antics. But usually this is a breeze comparing to what it used to be like.

But when he gets stuck in his old behavior, he is still completely unreasonable and provokes us very intensely. And it can last for a whole day. Oftentimes he gets "stuck," he is so strong-willed that sometimes he does not even know what to do. It could be that he wants a specific shirt that is in the wash and he still has to have it, or that he does not want to wash his hand before dinner. When we stop him or put limits he screams, "Stop it!"

When he was younger, he did not want to walk to daycare but insisted on riding in the trolley. Then when I put him in the trolley, he changed his mind and wanted to walk. Then he changed his mind again and wanted to ride in the trolley. And he would go on and on, and when I said, "Now I am the one who decides because I am in a hurry," the walk turned into a roaring conflict.

Also, he could ask for milk for breakfast, but when his older brother wanted water, Isak also changed his mind. Then we told him that first he had to finish his milk because he had asked for it. So then he turned his glass upside down and spilled the milk all over the table and the floor. Or when he decided that he did not want the food we had

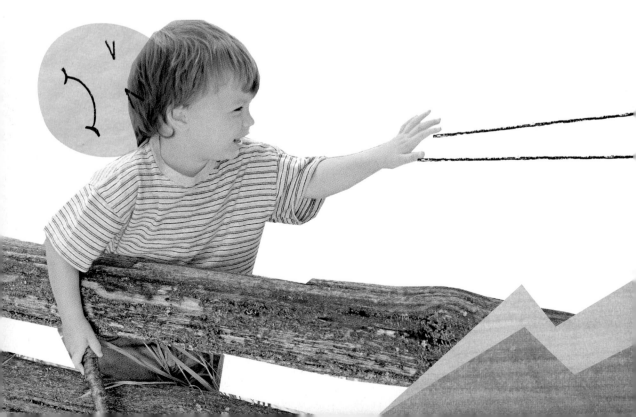

prepared, he would drop the plate on the floor. During the last year he has begun to learn to find compromises and he wants to be good, then we can point out what is about to happen and he will pull himself together. But sometimes he stills falls back, and things such as a meal can turn into a battlefield.

When Isak was about four years old, me and my wife were so exhausted and so distraught that we sought help at the Child and Adolescent Psychiatry Center. There we got some advice and insights that helped us move forward. But it is still incredibly hard sometimes. One of the big ordeals is to go off to daycare and the other one is to get him to go to bed. And then of course, the meal conflicts. At its worse, there is a fight about every little mundane detail and it is truly exhausting. Then everything must be done on his terms and conditions. The food must be threaded on the fork in a special way. When he has been to the bathroom he has to drink water before washing his hands. He has to have a tank top under his shirt, otherwise it all goes wrong. And when we refuse to agree to everything he wants he just screams. He is very sensitive to being controlled and hates to be rushed. If we rush him, he automatically gets bloody-minded. But in a family with children, every morning becomes a race against time. And by the way, no matter how much time we have, it is never enough anyway.

If we do not remind him and nag, he starts to play and forgets that he is going to daycare. And at night children have to go to bed at a reasonable time to be able to get up in the morning. But it is as if he wants and needs to prolong both the morning and the evening procedures. However, at daycare the teacher calls him a "fireman" for being so quick in getting dressed—this is something that Isak told us proudly himself. But he has to test us and finds it difficult to be a fireman at home, no matter the hurry we are in.

The hardest part of being a parent to such a demanding child is that we never feel pleased with ourselves. The worst was when he was smaller. Every day at work I would long for the boys and think that today I will not fall into the trap, today I will have infinite patience and we will be cozy together, just as we actually can be sometimes. But as soon as I get home, the misery begins. I want to be a wise and mature parent who manages the conflicts with my son. But every time there is a night or day fight, I get disappointed, thinking, "I could not do it today either." Then I feel like a miserable, worthless father. I try everything, but nothing works, and then I get totally frustrated.

Being consistent is not an option; instead I desperately try everything. I try to reason or I try persuading, I punish, I reward, I scream, I threaten and I force. Sometimes, for example, I hold him firmly and brush his teeth with coercion. Other times I give in and let him go to bed without brushing his teeth. Or I myself become like a toddler and stand there screaming and saying things that I am not proud of.

Nevertheless, I notice that the more "adult" I am able to be, the better it is. Especially in the last year, there has been a big difference. It is as if you become a child yourself when you are tired and provoked. The first three times you might manage to be pedagogical and calm, but if he has not been listening, then I know what kind of a day it is and all the previous conflicts fall upon me and it makes me tired, sad, and angry. "Not again," I think.

The only thing I have not done is to beat him. But sometimes I have been afraid of losing it, then I take him up to his room to give us both some space, but then he comes running after me. And sometimes when he has been extra difficult I have thought that I do not like him, that I do not want him. These are terrible and forbidden thoughts that I feel very guilty for. But the strength and joy runs out sometimes. It is fortunate that my wife and I feel the same way. Both of us feel equally helpless, despaired, and bewildered and can understand each other and talk about it. Isak challenges both of us, but sometimes his defiance is directed mostly towards me, and sometimes mostly towards my wife. It happens periodically but it can also vary the same day. When one of us is completely exhausted, we can hand it over to the other one and that is a rescue. Sometimes we wonder what we would do if we were single parents. How would we deal with life? But it is possible that things would not be quite as difficult then. When one of us is the only adult at home he becomes a little easier to deal with. It is as if he adapts his challenges to the possibilities. Although, there are of course exceptions to that as well. For a while we were worried about his older brother Samuel. At that time Isak was the one who ruled at home and the rest of us felt like extras. Isak's mood and strong emotions ruled all of us, and Samuel often came in second place. He was also tired of Isak's screaming and sometimes he would ask for earplugs. Quite often it also happened that Samuel "buffered" around Isak trying to help him in various ways so that there would be no more outbursts or conflicts. It felt very sad and this was probably one of the things that got us to ask for help from the Child and Adolescent Psychiatry Center.

One important thing we learned from there was to give Isak a break in the conflict sometimes. Before, the fights would often end with him weeping really badly with spurting tears and shouting "Love me!" But still refusing to do what he was supposed to, like brushing his teeth or getting dressed. But when Isak shouted "love me," he had given up, they said at the Child and Adolescent Psychiatry Center, and then he needed us.

103

We were advised to end the conflict at such times and take him in our arms. It was not all that easy when we ourselves were about to boil over with rage and were stressed, but when we have done it, it has worked better. We also got other advice on how we could change our own ways. Not only Isak, but we too were stuck in certain behaviors and reactions. We were advised to compromise more and to choose our battles, but also give him more resistance in some cases. They advised us to impose rewards and it has worked quite well. He gets a golden star if he has not said any bad words in three days and he gets to print Yu-Gi-Oh pictures on the computer when it has been a good day, and he likes that. Even Isak has learned to compromise sometimes. Perhaps because he has matured and gotten a little older. But it also helped that we parents have had help to understand him better. In recent times, we gave him the responsibility to get dressed on his own in the morning and it has worked out well. Then he is very happy and proud. The ambience at home has softened up a little bit and it is for the benefit of us all. Even Isak finds it difficult with all the fighting. Now, when things are calmer, sometimes after a day without any major conflicts he says, "Daddy, I did well today, right?" And he is really proud, then it feels wonderful to praise him. Isak has not had so much praise here at home. But what we have tried to do is to distinguish the fact that we do not like his behavior, but still, when things are quiet, really show him that we love him. And I am sure that he knows, and it is comforting to know that we at least managed to communicate this through all the conflicts.

We are of course also wondering why Isak is such a demanding child, but we have no explanation. We have asked ourselves whether we have done anything wrong and blamed ourselves. And yes, we have made lots of mistakes, but it turns out that all parents do, when you talk a little bit more seriously with them. So we do not think that it is our parenting that made him like this. Even when he was only three weeks old, his temperament could be sensed. He screamed and kicked intensely and powerfully, quite unlike his older brother. It is as if Isak was born with incredibly strong emotional expressions. He is not only the world's angriest but also the happiest, most charming, and most wonderful little boy.

About Klara, three years old: "The only thing that helps is me holding her"

Klara becomes like a wall when she decides on something; she has been this way from the beginning. She has always been spirited and energetic and has incredible integrity. You could say that once she has decided, the situation is hopeless. Her main weapon is a terrible scream. I often give in. Otherwise there will be at least half an hour of fighting.

Therefore, I choose my battles. As for clothes, I have given up. For a while, only nightgowns would do. Right now only a jean skirt will do. Dressing her up nicely is something I have given up on a long time ago. I do not interfere in her food choices either. I know she gets the nutrition she needs. She is not only angrier than other children but also happier. It is as if her emotions are extremely strong. She throws herself into my arms and shouts that I am the best mom there is and that she loves me. She is a very happy kid who charms everyone. She is early in everything; she started talking early and is very verbal. She has started to write letters on her own. Klara is quick-witted and always has an answer. Before Christmas, I said something stupid to her, that "If you are not nice, Santa will not come." Then she answered me, "So then Santa never comes to moms." The other day when she sat down in her older sister's chair she said merely, "Oh well Mom, now there will be a fight." But sometimes she surprises me. She always wants to press the flush button on the toilet and mercy on the one who does it. One day when I did it by mistake and got terrified, she said graciously, "I thought I would let you do it today, Mom."

When my limit is reached and I get really angry, sometimes Klara starts to cry. Then she cries as she shakes; she is completely heartbroken. Then, the only thing that helps is me holding her until she calms down.

She wants to decide at daycare as well. She rules the roost and is good at getting things going, she is liked by both children and staff.

Her older siblings think she is obnoxious, but they love her and defend her when I get angry at her.

Klara has always been strong and independent. She can answer for herself and speak up on how she wants things to be, and she is not at all shy or anxious. When she was two years old, she wanted to sleep over at the neighbors. Then she packed herself a toothbrush and other things she needed, followed the neighbor and slept there all night. She is not afraid to try new things; recently on a trip abroad, she rode an elephant alone, totally fearless.

Her dad died a few weeks before she was born. Sometimes I wonder if Klara's strength and integrity is associated in any ways with that. Perhaps she has been forced to be this strong and independent by the fact that I have been alone with the children. Sometimes I think I "fight" too little with her. But there is no use in it. It is difficult to defeat a strong three-year-old who has made up her mind. I hope reasoning with her will be easier when she is four years old.

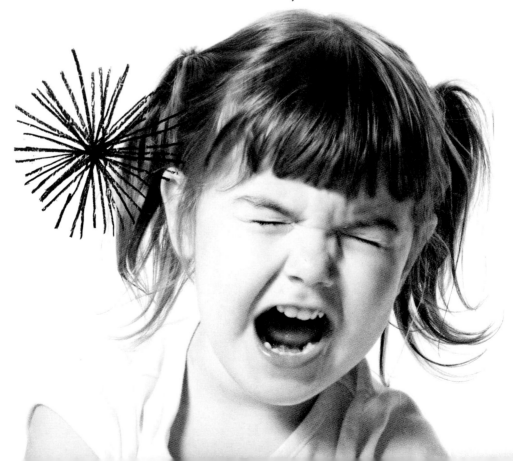

About Ellen, almost four years old: "She controls the whole family with an iron fist"

I am usually the one to take her to daycare. It is no cakewalk; rather, it's something that often makes me exhausted. Some mornings, it feels as if Ellen and I are fighting each other. She refuses everything: not these clothes, not these tights, no yoghurt, no chocolate, no brushing teeth, daddy cannot make the sandwich, the older sister should do it (who is in a hurry to get to school). Sometimes things are worse than usual.

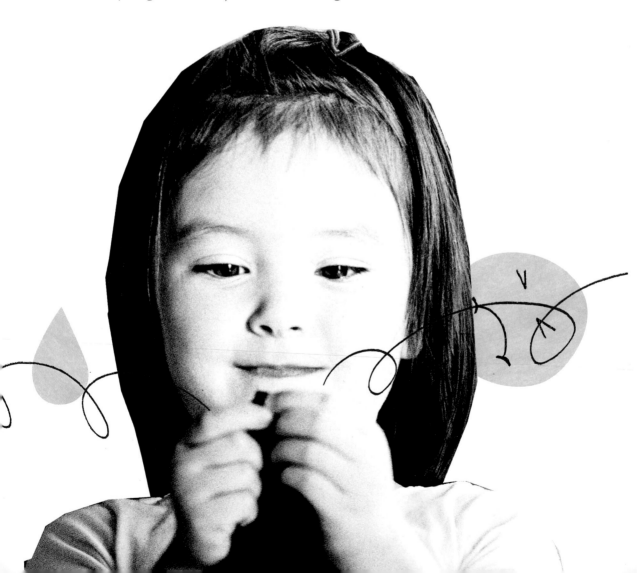

Sometimes, after endless unsuccessful negotiations, nagging, coaxing, and fighting, I have given up and, still in her pajamas, I wrapped a blanket around her and carried her, roaring, to the car. Then when we get to daycare I have been able to dress her in the car without any major problems before going inside. She probably thinks it is a little bit embarrassing to go to daycare in pajamas.

When things are at their worst, it does not matter how quietly we may do things in the morning. And finally I reach a limit. Partially, I feel the stress from work. Although it is true that I can somewhat control my hours, the later I get started in the morning, the longer the day I have to work. In the end, I end up annoyed. I get stomachaches and I feel that no matter what I do it never works out. Her sister who is a year and a half older also becomes worried and sad.

After a morning like this, when I am about to leave daycare, Ellen is sad and does not want me to leave. And I am also sad. Both of us have anguish because the morning is so difficult. I think she would have liked to go home with me to cuddle and make everything good again, and to be honest, this is exactly what I would like too. There are times when I cry out of powerlessness and despair after dropping her off. I feel like I've failed terribly. One time, someone from daycare kindly called me to tell me that Ellen calmed down and is happier than ever. Ellen and her older sister changed daycares about six months ago. It is a great daycare and the girls like it.

I also have my own experience about the fact that things can change quickly. When the children wake up, my wife has often already left for work so she can pick them up early. One morning, my wife was going on vacation and was at home when the children woke up and the morning chores began. However, she was busy getting ready for her trip. Ellen did not like that! And whatever I would do, she cried and screamed and shouted, "Let Mommy do it." Everyone in the family felt bad and no one could say a word to anyone; no one could talk over Ellen.

When mom was about to leave, Ellen ran and opened a small window where she could lean out and yell for mommy. I had to hold her so that she would not fall out. I am sure her desperate screams were heard several blocks away. But as soon as mom was out of sight, she paused abruptly and was as happy and as cooperative as ever. Ellen has always had a terribly strong will, she likes to make her own decisions and goes crazy if anyone else interferes. Oftentimes, it is as if she gets obsessions and gets stuck in them. I sometimes think that she understands it would be good for her to give in, to calm down, to let go of her obsession, but she cannot do it. I also feel that she is a very sensitive child who does not like to have her circles disturbed. That makes her anxious.

Her defiance was at its worst from ages two to three. Between three and four years old she became more "spoken" and then it became easier to understand her. Previously, in the "crises," it was difficult for her to speak and make herself understood, which probably contributed to her getting so angry. It being difficult to understand what she was saying when she was angry was of course frustrating for the rest of us in the family. She wanted – or did not want – something, but what? Now, when she is about to turn four, her mood has gone full speed again. Just when we thought she had calmed down . . .

Sometimes, we wonder if her strong defiance and her having to assert herself are due to the fact that our family is big and that she is the youngest of the siblings. Maybe she feels that she has to resort to shouting and defiance to make herself heard? It happens quite often that she tries to play the rest of us family against each other. However, I think that her older siblings are calm, kind, and tolerant towards Ellen, so I do not think she has to struggle so much to assert herself. Perhaps she is simply born strong, stubborn, and defiant.

Sometimes, we think we should have put more limits. But sometimes there is no time for it and it is difficult to be consistent. We resort to all possible solutions. Sometimes we try to talk to her. We plead, persuade, we try by hook or by crook, and of course by bribing her or attracting her with some kind of a reward. Other times we get angry and threaten her with retaliation. But once things go wrong, it does not really matter what we do because then she refuses anyway!

109

About Jacob, seven years old: "Jacob is not in a defiant phase; he is this way"

Jacob was a challenging child from the beginning. But we did not really understand that because he was our first child. We thought babies were like him. It was really only when Måns was born three years later that we understood how unusual Jacob is. As a baby he was incredibly alert, happy, and curious. He always wanted to be around us. Putting him on the floor or in the stroller was out of the question. He had to be carried, and only then was he pleased. I attended a couple of horrid mother meetings. All the babies lay on the floor and "talked" and flopped around happily while their mothers talked. Jacob wanted to sit in my lap and nothing else would work; he would just scream. It was tough with all the comments and good advice from the other mothers. They thought I was spoiling him. Jacob slept very poorly the first few years. It took several hours for him to fall asleep and Fredrik and I took turns to sit in his room until he had fallen asleep. In order to help him and prevent him from getting up, one of us would always sit in his room until he fell asleep. I have less patience than Fredrik and after a while I felt restless, I was sweating and feeling bad when I thought about everything else that had to be done in the evenings.

Once he fell asleep, he woke up about every hour. The first six months he would often wake up every twenty minutes. The first time that he slept through a whole night, he was three years old. It was crazy hard. The one who was going to get some sleep had to sleep in another room. Fredrik worked to be able to cope. At lunch he went down to the garage at his work, he loosened his tie and slept for forty-five minutes. This was his salvation. Jacob took such short naps that I almost never got to sleep during the day. I was exhausted, incredibly forgetful, and confused (and grumpy!) during this period. When I spoke to Child Health Center they said "You should have thought of this before you had children."

Jacob had – and still has – very high expectations of himself. He is afraid to make a mistake, everything has to be perfect and if it does not turn out like that he can break down. When he was only a year and a half years old, he dropped a vase on the floor and then he said, "God, how embarrassing." He was very premature and when he was two years old he learned the alphabet on his own. Then he told us that he could not fall asleep because he was annoyed with himself for not being able to remember some letter.

It was as if he had so much energy that he was not able to relax. He talked constantly and has a big need of moving around, a tremendous energy. We noticed that it helped somewhat if he was tired, so we encouraged physical activity. When he was two years old, I remember that he would cycle around the yard on his tricycle just before he would go lie down in the afternoon.

At age three, his sleep would gradually get better. But last year, when he was six, he had trouble falling asleep again. He could not relax but laid thinking about everything under sun – the solar system, the stars, how it all came to be and so on. It could take three, sometimes four or five hours for him to fall asleep. He has a little need for sleep but for us it was untenable that he was getting so little sleep, both for him and for us.

We tried every possible trick and method. (We tried the five-minute method when he was a year and a half or two years old.) Nothing worked. He would lay and worry about preschool and school. Eventually he got sleeping aid medicine for a period of time and it helped a little bit.

We have not had anyone to help us out us every now and then because our family lives elsewhere. We have not been able to keep babysitters because Jacob is so demanding.

As I said, it was first when Måns was born that we understood that Jacob is special. Having a child like Måns is a piece of cake in comparison; he was a baby-light. Måns slept for eighteen hours straight during the first period of time. When he was awake, he laid and looked around a little bit and "talked" to himself. The boys cannot be compared at any point. But even though they are different, they really

111

love each other. They are best friends and they hug and long for each other, and play together a lot. This is incredibly positive.

When he was three years old, Jacob's sleep was getting better. But he started to become more defiant. In the beginning we thought he was in a late defiance period, since he never had any two-year-old defiance, because he has always been incredibly "nice" and cooperative. But it just continued year in and year out. When he was six, we went to a psychologist who said, "Jacob is not in a defiance phase. He is this way." He is so strong-willed, he has an incredibly stubborn personality. He said no to everything from morning to evening. No to getting dressed, no to getting undressed, no to going to daycare, no to going home from daycare, no, no, no. He was so angry, sought conflicts, and could be defiant even when it came to fun things. One Sunday afternoon we were going to a swimming pool but Jacob was fighting about everything all the way there. Finally, we said that we were not going to go, because we cannot be in the swimming pool with him not listening or obeying. He had to choose between staying calm or staying at home. He chose to stay home, even though he loves to go swimming.

Other times he tried to provoke conflicts. He would behave rudely towards guests, scream at them they were stupid and that they should go home. He was so negative every time we did something he did not like or every time he thought something was wrong. One day, when he was four, he told a teacher at his daycare: "You should not be working with people because you do not like people. You should get another job." The teacher got so offended that she was crying when I came to pick him up. Something that has always been so contradictory with him is that, when he is in a good mood, he is incredibly nice, verbal, insightful, and incredibly fun to be around. We, our friends, and the teachers at daycare and at school share this opinion.

Obviously, we get angry at Jacob when he misbehaves. But if we get angry, he gets even angrier. Any pressure towards him causes back-pressure. But at times it has been difficult to cope with him. In the end, we felt that we could not do it. We felt like we were having a crappy life. It was not only about me and Fredrik, but also Måns was suffering because he had to be right in the firing line every night. So then we sought help from a psychologist. With the help and support from the psychologist we have eventually found a workable approach and started to accept Jacob as he is. We have stopped trying to change him and we stopped listening to all the well-meaning advice from everybody else that just made things worse.

It is only now that we have begun to accept that Jakob is like not like everybody else. Previously, we have stubbornly and desperately tried to force our round child into a square hole. But this is impossible and we know that now. Now we can love and appreciate him in a completely different way. In the past year we have also deliberately chosen a quieter life. Previously, both of us worked at least full-time and we commuted. Now, Fredrik reduced his hours by twenty-five percent. And I am now self-employed and can control my work and my hours on my own. We have completely eliminated stress from our lives, which has affected both us and Jacob positively. He is much more harmonious now. Another positive change is that Jacob started school. Preschool was hell for Jacob. He was saucy and questioned everything and thought it was extremely uninteresting. His teacher would throw him out or he went out on his own. In the evening he would tell us how he provoked his teacher. "Today I caused trouble because it was so boring that I did not want to be there." He spent that year in the coat room or the playroom, he did not participate in the classroom. And we spent endless hours on talking with the teachers, principals, special education teachers, and participated in class, but it did not lead anywhere.

At school, he has a teacher who understands him better and in the classroom, there is also a resource teacher because there are a number of troubled children in the class, so he helps Jacob and a few others too. But according to him, Jacob is doing so well now that he does not need a lot of support. This past year, Jacob made a lot of friends,

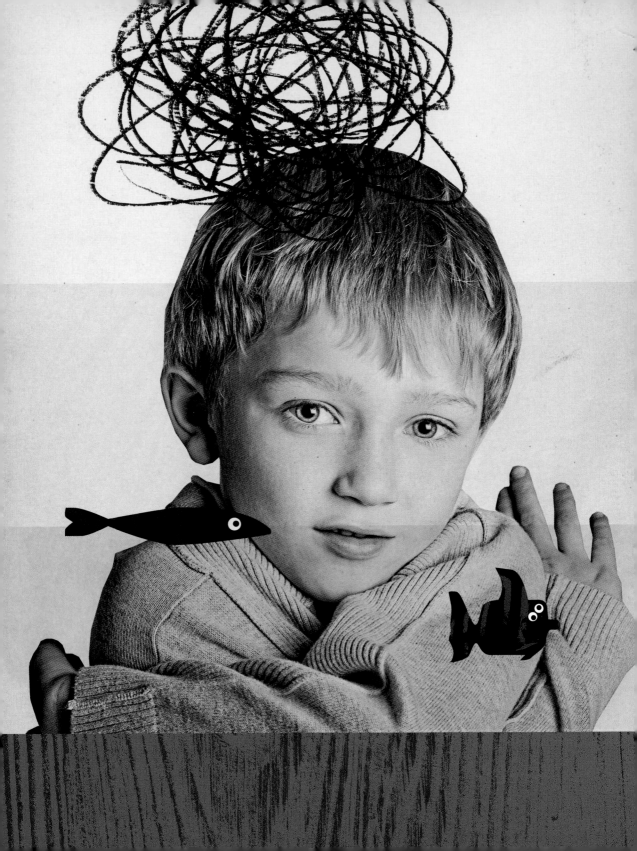

even if he does not have a best friend yet, which he longs for. Jacob is a soft guy, he is cowardly and not particularly "boyish." He paints and embroiders rather than playing football. He has been bullied by other boys. When he was younger he never participated in the games children his age played; he preferred to play with older children or the younger girl next door.

Another positive change for us is that my parents have retired. They live sixty miles away from us but we can see each other more often now and we can get the relief we need. Fredrik and I can go out and eat, do errands, or take a walk. On a couple of occasions we have also gone away for the weekend. In recent years, Jacob has spent a few summer days with my parents on their boat. They are fantastic with Jacob.

Jacob is a pretty serious boy. But if one does things with him that interest him, one can see the joy, the positive energy. One can see the wealth of ideas and desire. We try to encourage that and take him to the library and show him how he can find out things. He has become an expert on aquarium fish and it is amazing to see how important and positive it is for him to be an expert. He says "I do not need to be an expert on everything, fish is enough." Nowadays he can sit in his room and get involved in something. He needs peace and cannot be bothered with a lot of activities. Everything has really changed a lot over the past year. Jacob feels better and so do the rest of us in the family.

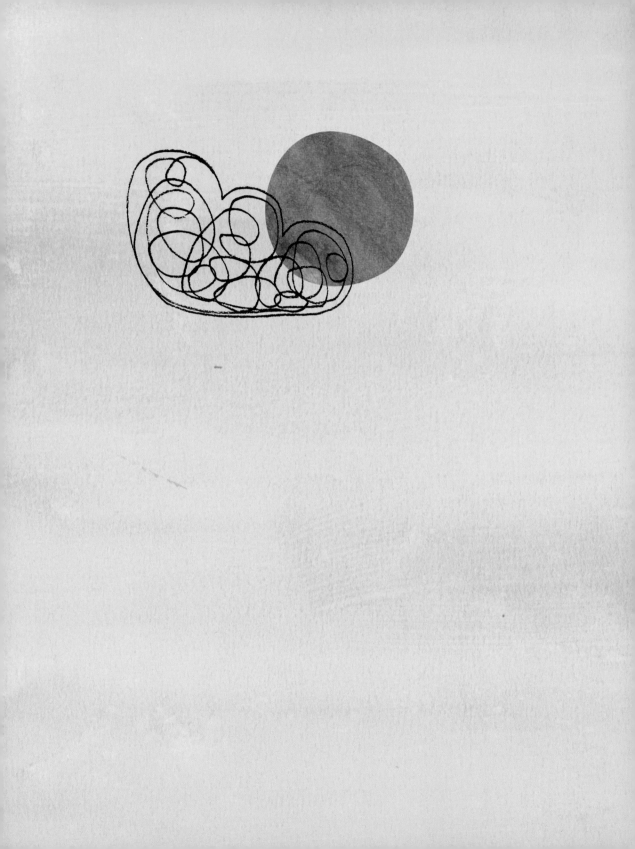

Around nine years old — the forgotten years

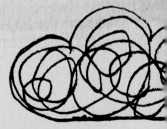

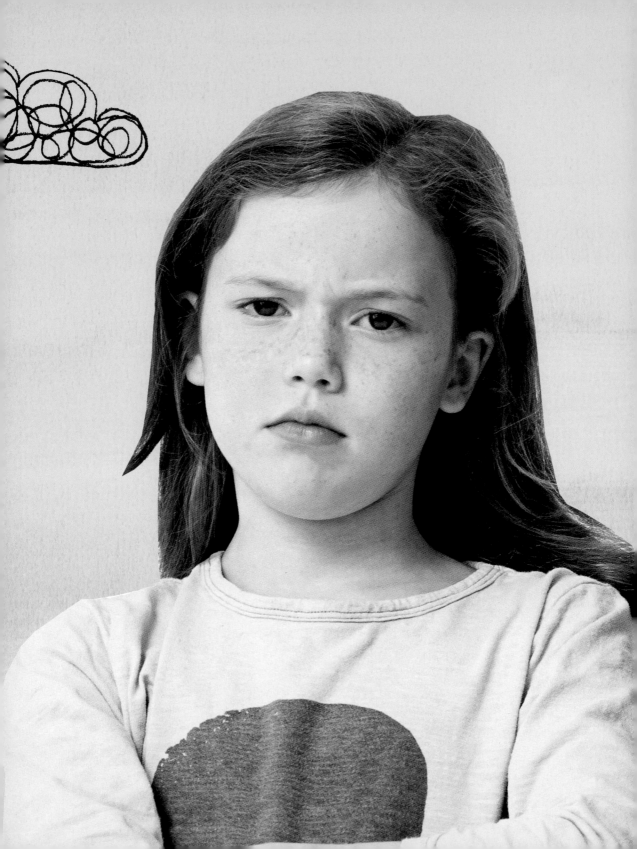

⋙→ AROUND NINE YEARS OLD – THE FORGOTTEN YEARS

AT NINE YEARS OLD THE child is vulnerable. It is normal that they are sensitive to criticism and assume that things will go wrong. The child is afraid to make a fool of himself and wants to be like everyone else. Self-esteem is often not at its peak. The nine-year-old is big and capable. But she also needs to be small and be hugged and cuddled with, and avoid having too-high demands.

Many nine-year-olds are a bit quiet and reserved and do not make much noise. Maybe this is why the years around age nine are called "the forgotten years." This is an age that has not been much researched or been of much interest. The nine-year-old crisis is different from the earlier periods of development. Then it was mostly about violent outbursts such as lying on the floor and screaming. Now it is a different kind of defiance, more introspective. But it can be just as tough, for both the child and the parents. As in all sensitive developmental stages, the child swings back and forth in time. They are both small and big. The child has a strong desire to get a grip on life and thinks about the big questions of life, about life and death, from where and to where. The child likes stability. Home should be as it has always been. But they are also curious about the outside world.

There can be some pretty fierce clashes at times, though in a different way than before. A six to seven-year-old can still lie on the floor and scream and fight with both arms and legs. But the nine-year-old has learned to use language and is good at making mom and dad speechless.

The adult world beckons and frightens

At nine years old, children begin to develop an interest in the adult world. Many, especially girls, are thinking more about their appearance, and they are interested in clothes and makeup. And last but not least, the child begins to become curious about the opposite gender, and sex. Parents can feel that the child is on their way into the adult world and that they are not needed in the same way. It is not unusual that the child occasionally spends a lot of time with friends and learns a lot about how life is in other families. The world expands and one understands that there are many different ways to live.

The child's self-awareness awakens in this age. They do not follow the adults' rules as they used to. The parents are not always the obvious authorities. The teacher is no longer an idol that the child obeys and follows, but someone they question and sometimes defy against. The child is curious and can argue. For the child, the adult world is not only something attractive. It can also be frightening, strange, and above all complicated. Now, the child has a need for introversion and pondering. It can be seen as an important preparation for puberty.

Knowledge is a great need. A nine-year-old can ask an endless amount of things and many learn

Matte, nine and a half years old

I lie a little bit and I am worried that I might get worse. If I have to be honest, I lie quite often actually. It has stuck, it has become like a habit. In order to hide that I lied, I lie a little more. If I almost did something I say I did not do it. When I get found out it does not feel good. It feels awkward.

120

how to find out about things on their own in books or online.

He likes to solve problems and is so constructive. The nine-year-old is thus busy with acquiring knowledge and pondering. No wonder that it can be a little difficult to get him to function in everyday life. It may require a lot of nagging to get him to eat breakfast and go off to school. The humor is different now compared to before, when there were a lot of pee and poop stories. The nine-year-old likes to tell stories and jokes and knows many by memory, but they are also much more "adult" than before. They have also learned how to use irony and understatement.

About Terese, nine years old

It is as if her self-esteem has become smaller, she has become less confident. At the same time she is sulky and grumpy, we can actually sense some teenage tendencies. She is not as anxious to please like she was before. And she has begun to care more about how she is dressed. She no longer shares everything with me. She sits in her room and writes letters and I do not know what is in them.

The environment becomes increasingly important

Now, many children get to start practicing how to move around in the community, go to the library and get to the dance, get to the soccer practice or the theater group, all on their own. Maybe they can take the bus to grandpa and grandma or go to town and buy a birthday present for the party they are going to.

For the child it may be a big step and an effort to cope with things that are obvious for us adults. Many elements are to be managed and in the correct order. They should pack fruit, remember the gym bag, bring money and the bus pass, go home at the right time, wait for the green light, take the bus in the right direction, change to another one (the right one!) and get off at the right bus stop, find the gym, lock the clothes in the locker, keep track of the locker key, not forget the jacket, and so on.

About Jenny, nine and a half years old

She has always been a confident, happy, and stable girl. And then, six months ago, she suddenly lost her foothold. She oscillated between being small and big. She sought for my closeness, snuggled up in my lap and cuddled and told me she felt lonely and that she thought she was useless.

Then, she would suddenly become distant and scream and be mean to me. She accused me and did not want to see me. I did not know how to respond to her because no matter what I did, it was all wrong. After some time, it slowly improved and now she is in a quiet period again.

But coping with such things strengthens confidence and opens up the world a little more each time. Children at this age are heavy consumers of television, movies, computers, and games. They watch both children's and adult programs and maybe show an interest in reality shows. They want to choose what to watch and they watch mostly alone, with no adults around. These are obvious and important parts of most nine-year-olds' lives, both to gain knowledge and training, but pleasure too, of course.

But there are disadvantages too. On the one hand, there can be too much sitting still. We know today that children move too little, that even children of this age are "couched." And on the other hand, studies have shown that television and movies can be scary and make children anxious and fearful. A third disadvantage of too much watching TV and playing video games is that the children have much too little time to play on their own.

All this causes a lot of nagging and quarrels in the family. Even though we do not feel that nagging and fighting is of any help, we should still do it, because then at least we make the children feel guilty and then, at the best, they will not sit as long in front of the computer or TV. Parents and children need to make up rules together on times and how long they are allowed to be seated. Then, when time is running out we must warn the children about it.

To belong

Children at this age are still good at playing. They like to dress up and can organize theater performances. They can play intense fantasy games that can last for hours, or even days. One mother said that her nine-year-old played the same fantasy game for months. They developed the game day by day; it grew and changed, but basically it was the same game.

Children around nine years old often play in groups of two or three but also in larger gangs. Who is the best friend or who is in the gang can change fast. There are sudden disagreements and then everybody is friends again just as fast. Nine-year-olds like huts and secret nooks and clubs, often with rituals that are only for the initiated. Secret languages and codes are also common. Spending the night in a tree house, barn, or a tent is the height of happiness, even though it is possible that the children come home late at night.

Children play happily in nature by damming up the creek, building sand castles, climbing trees, catching crabs or tadpoles, walking the tightrope and arranging jumping competitions. They are good at organizing these games and they can come up with the most complex regulatory systems. There may be long moments of drawing straws or doing eenie meenie miney moe over who gets to start the game.

It is important to have friends, to belong to a group and be accepted there. They engage with zeal and fervor. It can be very difficult not to be "approved" in the circle of friends, or not to be part of the soccer team. Nine-year-olds can be quite mean to each other. "You can join, but not you." It is important that everything is fair, both towards friends and at home among siblings. Nine-year-olds find it easy to feel unfairly treated and they carefully make sure that everything is done properly. Boy and girls often play apart. But they also play together in smaller and larger groups.

Anders, nine years old

Adults are often bothersome because they misunderstand what happens between children without knowing the background of it. It can be so wrong. If we fight among friends, they always have to get in the middle of it and say let's forget about it, now you are friends again and let us do something else now. That makes you so very angry! They do not even know what happened, why we quarreled in the first place.

About Sofia and Helena, age nine

My twin girls spent the entire summer playing with their pretend horses in the neighboring farm. The horses had their own stall with nameplates in the barn. The horses were given hay, water and treats. They were taken out for jumping competitions and shows. The girls never got tired, the game continued for many weeks. They knew very well that it was imaginative, but they got very offended if we did not play along in the game and took the horses seriously. At the same time, they got embarrassed if we told others about their game. Then, the game suddenly became embarrassing and childish.

For some, soccer, hockey, or dancing is an important element in life. This is where they have an outlet for their energy and this is where friends are.

Their music plays an increasing role in the nine-year-old's life. It can be on for hours and at high volume. This is a small taste of teenage life. Many nine-year-olds dream about having their own animal. But soft toys are also needed; they still fulfill and important function.

Wild mixing

Many children read a lot when they are around nine years old. Some disappear into the world of books to such an extent that they hardly notice what is happening in the environment. When the child finds a writer they like, they can go through a whole series of books in a short time or reread books. One mother told us that her son read *The Brothers Lionheart* eight times in a row. Reading aloud from an exciting book is appreciated by most children. It creates unity and can be the stage for an exciting conversation.

Most can mix children's books with books for older people, "junk books," comics, and high-quality literature. Other children read only comic books. They think that books are boring. Many nine-year-olds also mix all kinds of TV shows, everything from qualified literary programs to reality shows and competition programs. They assimilate everything that can teach them about how adult life works.

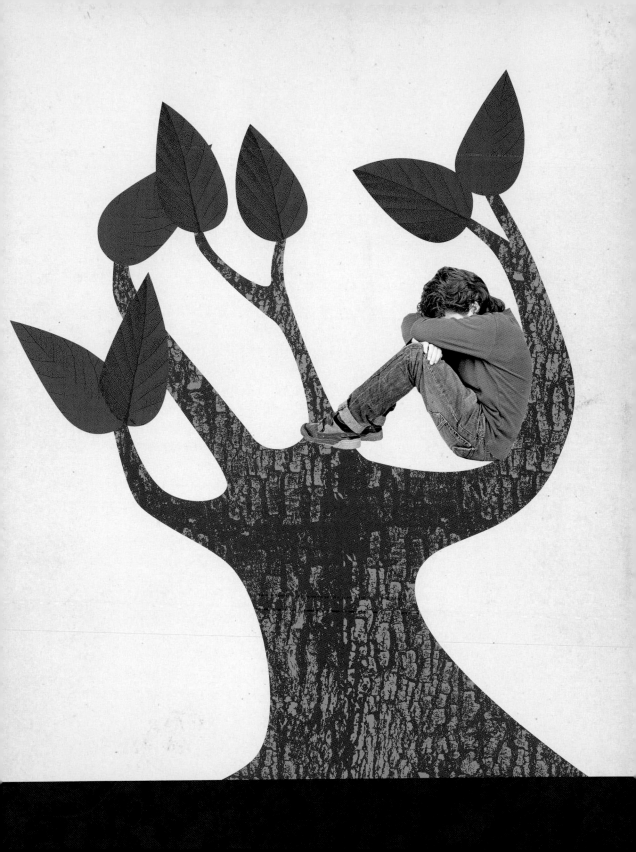

Many do not feel well

Thoughts about life and death, why we live and why we die often occupy the nine-year-old. It is not uncommon to have dark thoughts which take various physical expressions such as stomachaches, headaches, and nausea. School nurses tell us that there is a huge rise in the number of visits to their office at ages nine through ten. Studies show that the number of behavioral problems and symptoms increase dramatically at this age. Every fourth nine-year-old has some form of mental symptoms. It may include aggressiveness, passivity, fear of separation, difficulty in sleeping, introversion, anxiety, and depression. The child may feel alone and excluded.

Reading and writing difficulties often occur in this age. Especially boys may find it difficult to follow the teaching in school and they can be disruptive in class. Some say that the aggressive and unruly behavior is in fact a sign of sorrow rather than anger. Studies show that boys show more aggression and insensitivity, while girls often become worried and get anxious when others in the class fight.

For the child it obviously feels frightening and worrying to be in the midst of an intense developmental period, with all the symptoms that may be present and all the problems that may occur both in school and at home. Children at this age need to be alone with their thoughts and secrets. Interacting with a nine-year-old requires tact and consideration.

Between ages nine and ten, many children often consider the big issues of life: life and death, war and peace, love and hatred, health and illness, grief and regret, joy and sorrow, justice and injustice, history and future. The child also thinks a lot about who he is and how he is perceived by others. He is a seeker who is about to find his own identity. He is a brooder who is easily gripped by discouragement and anxiety.

Kajsa, nine years old

I often think about death. I believe that when someone dies, they go to heaven if they believe in God. Sometimes I believe in it and sometimes I do not.

126

The child realizes more and more what it means to be an adult with responsibilities and obligations. They can compare their own situation with that of others, and can be both sad and angry if they feel that they are worse off than others. But the child not only needs to be alone. She also has a great need to talk with adults about her thoughts and feelings, both with parents and with others, such as teachers, after school camp staff and sport coaches.

Divorce

When the child is nine years old, quite a number of children have separated parents. The separation might have happened long before, but now the child knows more about the adult world and about adult relationships. Thus, the child now understands better what it means and thinks about things like guilt and responsibility and how he will cope with his own relationships in the future. Many choose an alternate living after a divorce. This works well for most children who then get to keep a close daily contact with both parents. The disadvantages of

Mattias, nine years old

The worst thing about divorce is when they hand us children over to the other parent on Sunday evenings. They hand over the bags, and me and my little sister. Then you feel like a thing. When I told Mom about this yesterday, she said that they will stop handing us over like that, but we will instead go to school from her place on Monday morning and then go to Dad's place after school on Monday afternoon. I actually think this is much better.

things being in the wrong place, for example, tend not to be a major problem.

For the child it is of course positive if mom and dad can cooperate in a good way. This gives the child important knowledge about relationships. But it is almost inevitable that a divorce entails a lot of sorrow and anger, and for a certain period of time even feelings of vengeance between the parents. The first year is almost always chaotic and tough for everyone, a year of grief. The child can understand and handle this, if the parents then begin to work together better.

THINGS TO CONSIDER

→ The child is vulnerable and sensitive although not as aggressive as before.

→ The child is both big and small, and they need to be both. It is important to "be right" — not to treat the child as a toddler when they need to be treated in a more adult way, but at the same time not putting too many requirements on their shoulders. Both openness and responsiveness are required in order to manage this balancing act.

→ The child needs their parents, although it may seem like the opposite. "Go away" can mean "Come."

→ Be aware of psychosomatic symptoms. Many nine-year-olds have stomachaches, headaches, sleep disorders, or feel sick because they do not feel completely fine mentally. It is important to address these problems before they grow too large.

→ Some parents worry when their children read only comics and "junk," but all reading provides good reading training and is positive, experts agree.

→ Reality shows and competition shows can provide children with much knowledge of the adult world and could become the basis for fun and good discussions, especially if you watch them together.

→ A child who is involved in a divorce at this age needs to talk about the separation. But it may also be necessary if the divorce occurred before. Perhaps only now the child is mature enough to discuss what happened.

→ It can be liberating for the child to be told that it is both common and normal to be sad and worried at this age. Time for serious talk about life's issues is therefore needed. But nine-year-olds also need time for regular, casual get-togethers with mom and dad. Playing games, cooking, skating together, taking trips or going to the movies.

→ Determine how the child will live after a separation, so she does not feel that the parents are leaving her out.

→ Explain why and talk about how things will be if there will be any major change in the family, such as relocation or separation.

→ Be aware of school truancy and bullying, both victims and bullies.

USEFUL READING

Julia's Book by Helena Dahlbäck.

Concerning Love & Mathematics by Anna-Karin Eurelius.

A Small Book about Malin by Ylva Karlsson.

Hedvig and Hardemos Princess by Frida Nilsson.

Divorce, Children and Parents by Malin Alfvén and Kristina Hofsten.

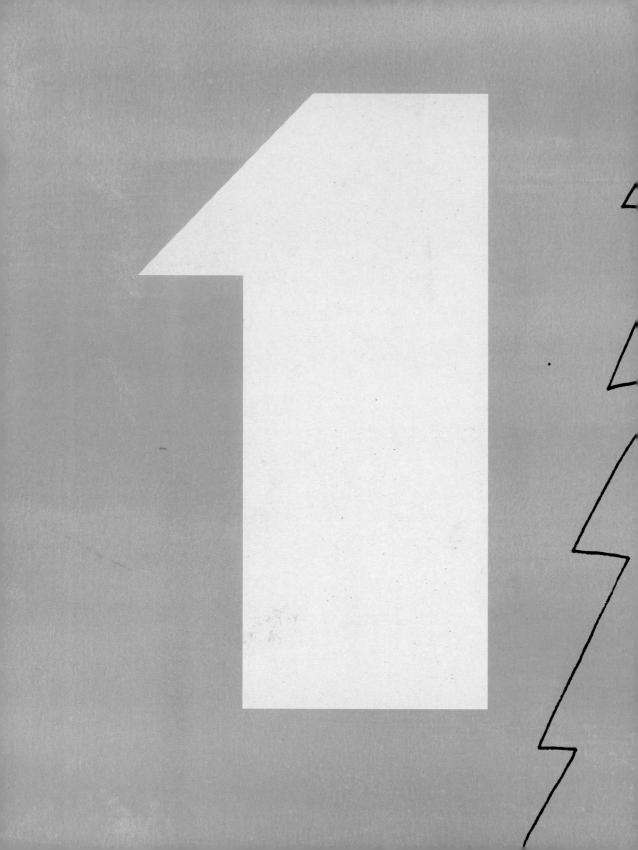

2

Twelve years old – a period of transition

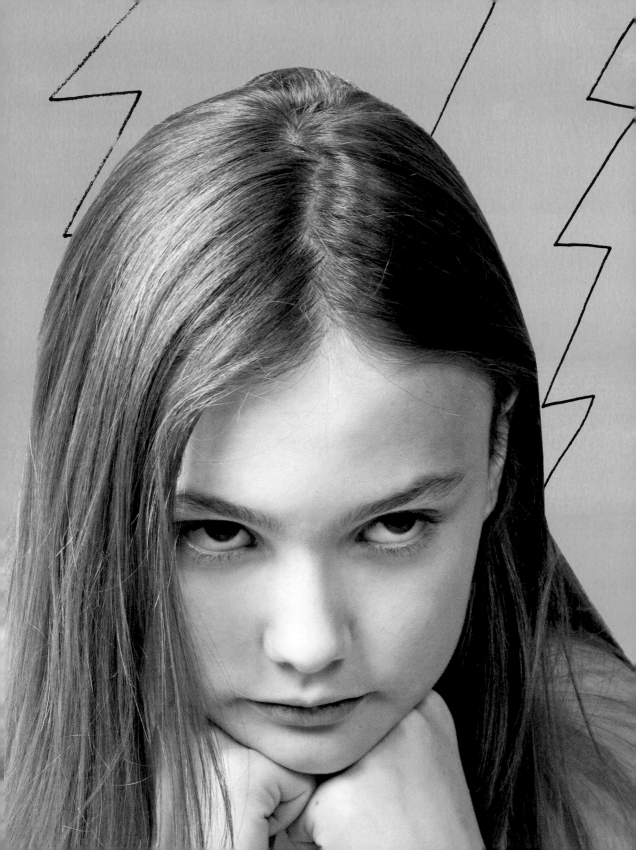

MANY TWELVE-YEAR-OLDS start to prepare for adult life by taking more and more interest in their appearance. The child that you almost had to force into the shower is now difficult to get out of the shower. Before a party, they can try on clothes, makeup, and hairstyles for hours. But the twelve-year-old still has a lot of child in her and needs to play childish games. Sometimes it may be difficult to understand that the twelve-year-old also is a child. Just like the children try on different looks, they also try on different attitudes. For us parents, it can be tricky to be on the right level of expectations. It is now that we often call other parents and look for support

Too small and too big

As a parent, you get accustomed to it being a roller-coaster. Curse words are common and you might be told to go to hell. Everything the parents do is wrong, crazy, stupid, and worthless. But sometimes the children will come and seek comfort, hugs, and cuddling. The child who just despised everything that mom was, in the next moment listens with great seriousness and pays attention to what she says. It can be difficult to find the right balance, to follow the abrupt changes.

133

The child can be tough and distant. It can obviously be difficult for the parent to be so questioned, especially if their own self-esteem is not very good. Recently, the child was a positive ten or eleven-year old who did question, but still admired and loved his parents unconditionally. Now, the parent is just completely wrong! Wrongly dressed, having wrong opinions, saying stupid things, and being dorky when friends are at home. It can be difficult to fall from an admired idol to a recipient of open contempt.

If it is any consolation, it is probably even more difficult for the child to have these powerful emotional storms. Then you have to withstand and trust your parenting skills and realize that you are the main support for the child – even though it does not seem to be so in every moment. It is not so easy for the twelve-year-old to keep up with the parents' approach. One is either too small or too big, twelve-year-olds may complain.

"You are too big to behave like a toddler." "You are too small to be out late at night." The child is big or small whenever it suits the parents. All twelve-year-olds do not react equally though. Some are unusually strong and extroverted, others are more sensitive and introspective.

About Tove, twelve years old

You have to keep up. She loves to dress provocatively with a bare belly and mini skirt, jewelry and makeup. But then all of a sudden she is a child. She puts a pillow on the banisters and she pretends to be riding it like a horse, much like something a four or five-year-old would do, and she wants us to watch. This contrast between teenager and childish games is too hilarious. But of course, we play along and ask if the horse has been fed.

134

Private room

There are twelve-year-olds who prefer to be alone, who mostly engage in the computer or reading. There are children who are true readers and read wherever they are. It is common for twelve-year-olds to engage completely in a certain interest, such as constructing something and learning everything in a special area. But most are very social, they surround themselves with many friends. Above all girls often have a close best-friend-relationship. The opinion of friends is the most important. The goal is to be popular and well liked. It is not very unusual that twelve-year-olds shoplift, make graffiti or something similar to impress their friends and to be accepted in the gang.

A private room or a private corner is something that twelve-year-olds appreciate; they want to be able to withdraw and lick their wounds as needed. They like to be alone with their thoughts and try on clothes and hairstyles without any comments from parents and siblings. They need a space to be undisturbed with their friends. A sign on the door saying "Private Area" or similar is almost a rule.

The twelve-year-old likes to claim his territory, screaming "Get out, I was here first!" to his siblings if they happen to come into the living room or the kitchen when she was there first. But the awkwardness and the need to be alone is just one side of the twelve-year-old. He needs his

About Klara, twelve years old

We have a "girly" and close relationship, Klara and I. We go out shopping together and borrow each other's clothes. We often go to the movies together and can talk about everything, we have a lot of fun together. But sometimes Klara likes to be alone. She suddenly becomes quiet and withdraws to her room. She is still not openly distancing herself from me, but I suppose it is coming. I remember how I was in that age. I loved my Mom but I could not help mocking her and saying mean things to her, making her really sad. Then I had terrible guilt, and we reconciled and became friends again.

135

**About Albin,
twelve years old**

I like being twelve. It's just the right
age. I'm not big or small, just in between.
I like having more responsibility than I had
before. I am not a teenager yet, but I have
seen and heard what a hassle it can be.
Being in between can be a disadvantage,
too. I can't do some things because I'm
too small and I shouldn't do some things
because I am too big.

family and likes to socialize, but on his own terms. He starts tugging the strings holding him back, but is still not yet ready to cut them.

The big questions of life

It is common for children in this age to think a lot about the meaning of life and death. They are not only here and now, but also form part of the universe and eternity. They ponder over good and bad and injustice. Why should some people be born into hunger and misery while others live in abundance and luxury?

They have a strong sense of justice and can be upset about people being unjustly sentenced, prisoners executed, mistreated animals. The twelve-year-old may even take up strong opinions and become an animal rights activist, a vegetarian, or join a peace movement. Maybe they think that their parents have "wrong" opinions and criticize them harshly. But at the same time, they need their parents as an interlocutor and sounding board. Many even take great pleasure in talking with other adults, such as relatives, a leader, or the parent of a friend. Discussing life issues in depth with a twelve-year-old is a privilege.

Twelve-year-olds dream about their future; they fantasize about different professions, whether they will fall in love and have children. Everything is a preparation for adult life.

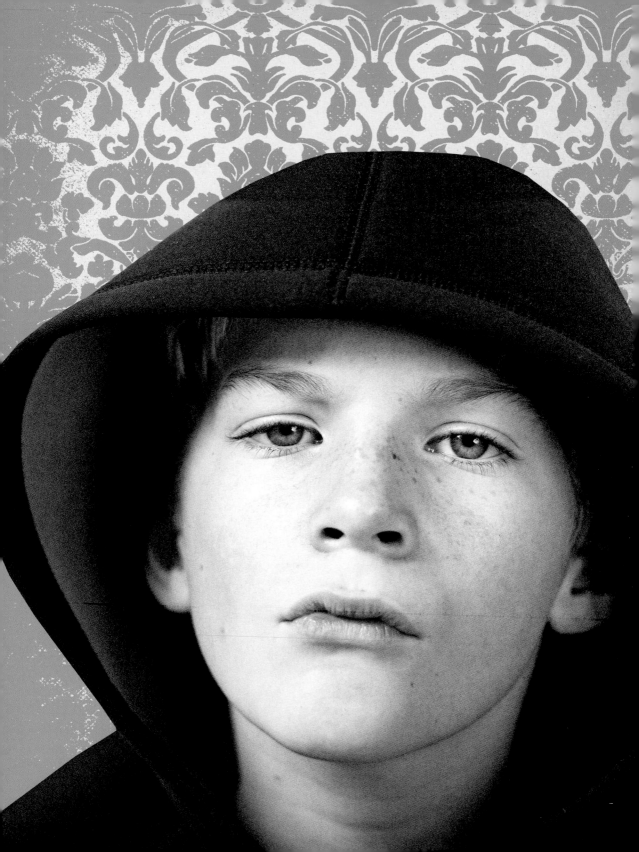

THINGS TO CONSIDER

→ The twelve-year-old is in a borderland, is both small and big. Show your child respect both when they need to be independent and adult, and when they need to be small and needy.

→ Implement the right kind of requirements at the right time.

→ Give yourself time to talk to the child, both about everyday things and about the big questions of life.

→ Respect the fact that the child needs to be left alone, to have their "own space." Do not intrude. Do not read diaries. Respect the signs on the door, but be there when your child needs you.

→ Let your twelve-year-old find his way to his style without too many comments about things such as makeup, hairstyle, and clothing.

→ Do not accept the child saying mean and despicable things to you. Tell the child that these are things one may think but should not say.

**About
Sara, twelve
years old**

Now she pulls away so clearly from her younger siblings. She shuts herself in her room, alone or with other girls, and wants to be alone. She tries on clothes and makeup, wants to try on different styles and tries to find her own. She can be on the phone for hours, she goes to parties on the weekends and devours soap operas. On weekends, she walks around in her pajamas all day long.

USEFUL READING

Jerker by Helena Axelsson Östlund.
King Steve's Luminous Hip Hop Bible by Thomas Fröhling.
The Flea and the Ice Princess by Kerstin Gavander.
Far From Cool by Ingrid Olsson.

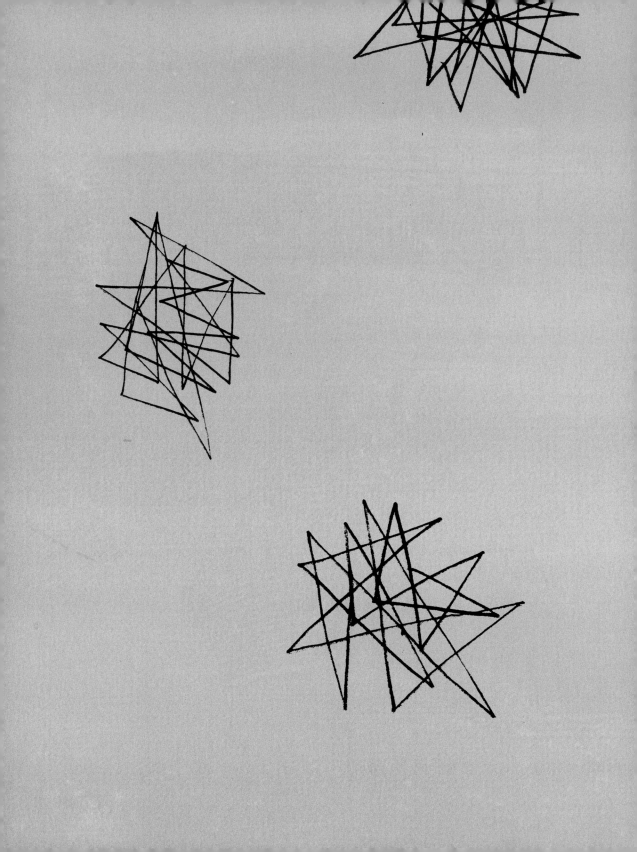

Adolescence — goodbye to childhood

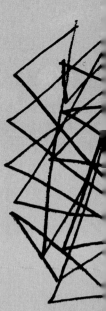

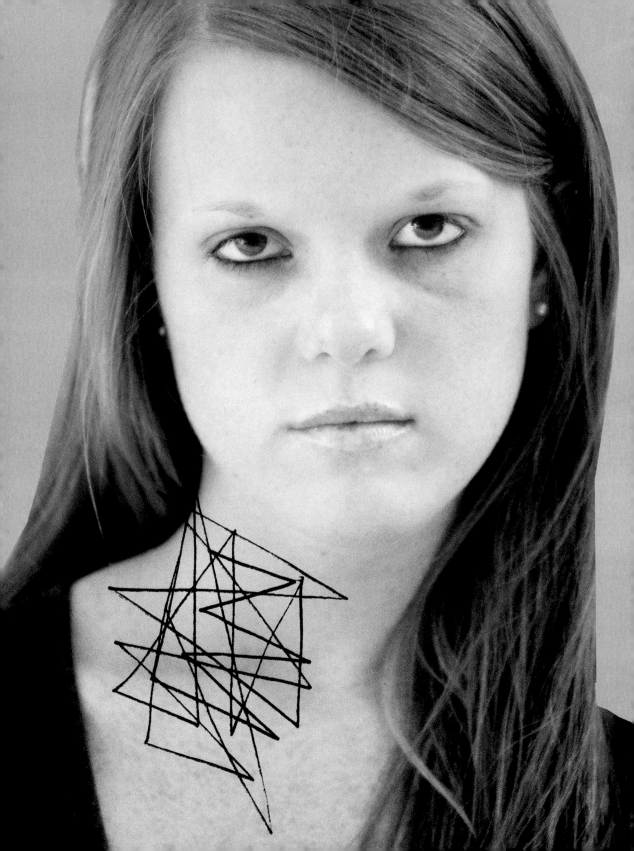

PUBERTY MIGHT BE the most intense defiance period in the life of many. This is the period when we leave childhood and gradually move into adulthood. When we are in a shorter or longer period of struggle with the rest of the world and ourselves in order to develop and be able to move on in life. How this development might be, what kind of problems may arise, and how one as a parent can understand and manage these developmental crises that might occur during adolescence is not the topic of this book. But we have included a story written by Malin Hägglund. She wrote it when she was nineteen and had vivid memories of how it felt to be a lost, insecure, and defiant teenager.

Who loves a teenager?

Who loves a teenager with a bad posture and a listless gaze? Who, other than her parents? A teenager with body parts growing out of step – nose, hips, belly and breasts, nothing is in unison. Everything is askew and growing pains are almost visible on the outside. Pimples soaking under greasy bangs on the forehead, pores producing sebum that becomes an oily coating that polishes blackheads until they shine.

143

Powder and concealer leave behind superfluous layers, so thick that they burst onto the skin. Orange, beige, and suntan-colored: all grotesquely unbecoming on a winter-pale face. The sad part is that all this lubricating and covering shows even more clearly that the person is ashamed and wants to hide something.

Thighs and stomach, once of a child, are now just pure fat – did all of this happen overnight? Lucky is the one who is skinny as a punk rocker. Who loves someone who hates to be in their own body?

As if all of this were not enough, there is also a huge mess inside. The inside of a person reflects the disharmony on the outside. Or the opposite is more reasonable: The outside reflects the inside. Who loves someone who believes, no, someone who *knows* that she has the answers to the big questions? The humility shown before these questions by the parent-generation can only mean one thing: she, merely fourteen, must be a genius, is it not so?

She obviously dresses in black, just like the big artists, and locks herself in the girl's room. There, she feels big emotions, the biggest there are to feel. How much can a human body take? When does the heart break?

She keeps a journal and writes poetry, paints in oil, and listens to music. She drowns in melancholy and somewhere in midst of all the pain and discomfort, she enjoys herself excellently. She has her friends, she certainly does. But they seem to be preoccupied with themselves and their own transformation. For some, it has yet not started, so with them their friendship must slowly die on its own. Everyone develops differently and relationships are so fragile, so fragile.

A small hormonal swing leads to a sudden and dramatic outburst that becomes the end of that friendship. Detest and hate, so long and good bye.

Who wants to stand next to someone who resembles a tangled ball of knots? With uncertain movements, nervous glances, hand sweating, and palpitations. Who loves a small one with a broken soul, a seeker who fumbles around, lost and blind? Who loves a loser?

144

If you have a child, a small child who will become big, prepare yourself for a change. You have a little kid with pink cheeks who jumps up out of bed each morning and sings about a new and wonderful day. Can you in your wildest imagination see a future beast in her? The most erratic and hypersensitive piece of human being. If you can, can you also see something else in your teenager, something powerful and good?

Imagine that you are unreasonably pleased with your fourteen-year-old's outburst, of her at least not being indifferent. Be glad that she at least does not have the goal of becoming *Miss Sweden* and for not doing drugs, at least not yet. If you take her thoughts and words very seriously, her ill-founded statements about injustice and politics, as if she was a professor of political science, if you show her respect, maybe the process can be somewhat relived and lead to a smoother transition from child to adult?

Soon she is fully grown and will be moving out. Take care of these quivering years. Be a rock, a calmness, and an example. Someday she will hopefully come out on the other side, strong, brave, and beautiful. The pain and confusion must have a meaning and be necessary for a better and freer life. It has to be this way because I cannot stand the thought of anything else.

Malin Hägglund

USEFUL READING
Trust Your Teen by Ingegerd Gavelin

145

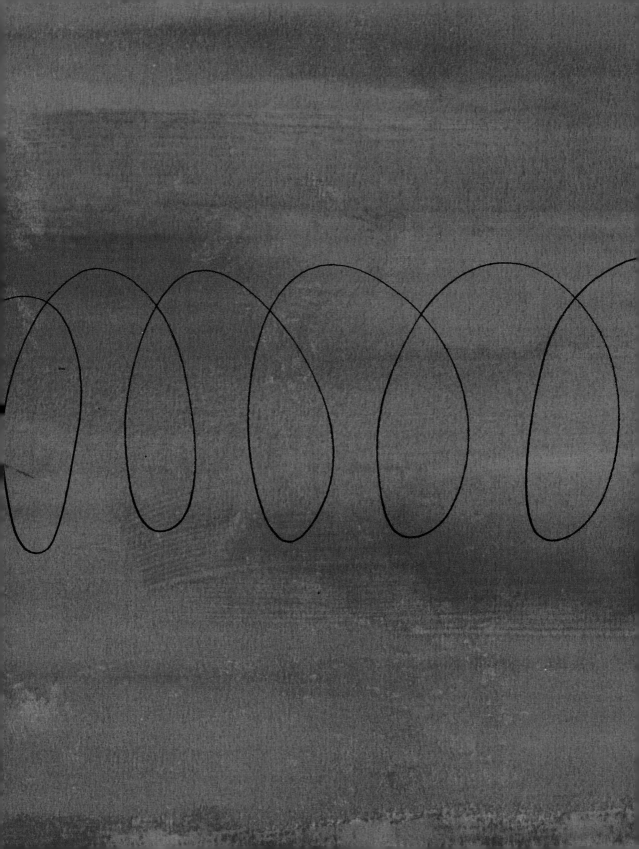

Pregnant – something entirely new

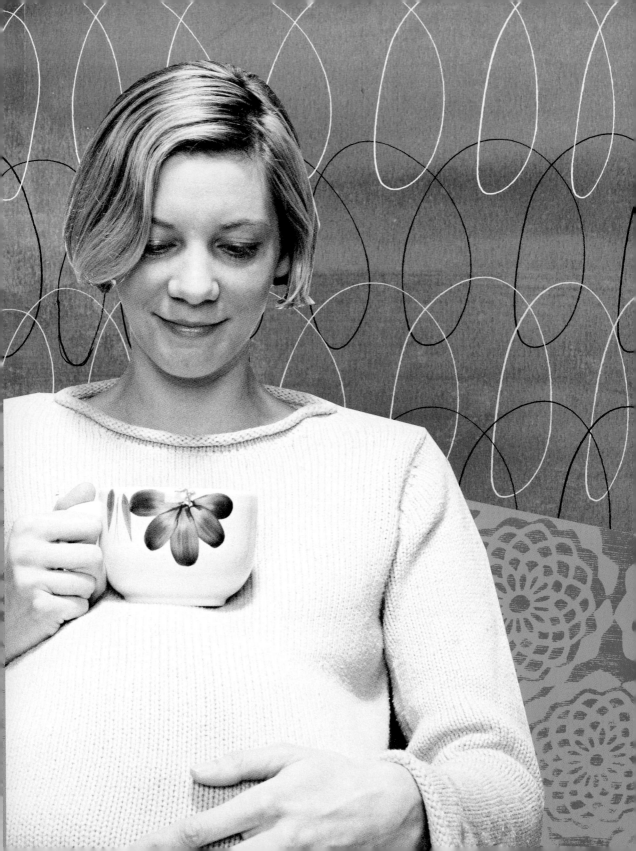

TO BE IN THE OBSTINATE age surely belongs to childhood, right? No, one can be defiant one's whole life when something big and life-changing happens. Pregnancy is one of the most tumultuous periods in adult life, it is also a time of maturity and development – and defiance. That goes for the future mother, but also for the man who is about to become a father. This is a time when we go back and reflect upon our own childhood and our own parents, and how we are as people. We question, think of how it was and how it will be. It is also common to think about death. During pregnancy, we think about the new, the unknown. What about delivery? What will the child be like? How will it look? How are we going to be as parents? Old wounds can be torn open. But we also get closer to intense feelings of happiness, and good memories pop up. We simply get closer to our emotions than otherwise. In this way, we approach the baby's way of being.

The one who expects pregnancy to be a walk on delightful clouds is often disappointed. Most women feel more or less bad, at least periodically. They can have serious, anguished thoughts, and may feel sick and be very tired and have trouble sleeping. And then it is possible to feel like a failure, because you are supposed to be happy. But the

149

Emma, twenty-five years old

My child will be born in a few weeks and I am getting more and more worried. The childbirth is around the corner and I must go through it, whether I want to or not. And I have no idea how it will be or how I will cope with the pain. I cannot change my mind, this almost gives me a sense of panic. It has not felt really real before. I have been happy and felt good. But now it feels mostly scary.

feelings of concern and anxiety play an important role in life. They help us to mature as people and develop into good parents. Being pregnant is something entirely new. It is obvious that the mother-to-be sees herself and her childhood in a completely new way than before.

Preparing for the unexpected

Expecting a baby is to prepare for the unexpected. It is a period in life that we have no control over. We cannot control the baby. You can be your usual self, but you have a little person inside of you who controls your life. And becoming a parent might not be as you had imagined at all. Some people do not worry so much about what will happen but take each day as it comes. Others are more concerned about the unexpected. They prefer to know exactly what will happen, how it will happen and when it will happen.

Then it can be especially difficult to be pregnant, since it is something we actually cannot have full control over. There are those who take six ultrasounds, for example. The more knowledge, the less anxiety. Others prefer to be prepared for the unexpected and are not interested in ultrasounds and amniocentesis.

Nowadays, many find out the sex of the child in order to be prepared. Others do not want to know the sex of the child but want to keep their surprise. Having children means to change and this takes courage. It is a challenge and a way to mature.

Nine months of pregnancy is needed for us to have time to prepare. This is one of the reasons for why it is so hard to have a miscarriage, because it intervenes in the predestined. Although we know there might be a miscarriage, that the baby can be born too early, and that the baby might die at birth. But we automatically prepare for an end date and it feels overpowering if the baby comes too early or if we go over time.

Even a few weeks too early can feel like a strike against you. Going into labor a few weeks, or maybe months, too early can feel like a disaster; we have not had time to fully prepare ourselves.

Adoptive parents know from the beginning that there is no given time when they will get the baby. They live with uncertainty and therefore need to cope with it. But once they get a date for when the baby is to be picked up, it feels incredibly frustrating if there are any changes in the plans. And if for some reason one does not get the awaited baby, the grief becomes heavy. The love for the child has already begun to grow even if you have only seen the child in a photo.

Gunilla, fifty years old

When my daughter became pregnant she wrote me a long letter. She wrote about events form her childhood which she was not "done" with, and which she had the need to talk about. There were some really difficult things that suddenly appeared in her mind. Mainly, it was things concerning the relationship with her biological father and her stepfather, my husband from that time. She felt I had not been there for her when the relationship with her father became difficult.

At first I felt a reluctance to bring up these old things. I was defensive and defended myself. But I realized that it was important to her. We talked a lot about the past, and it felt as if it was necessary for her, but it was good for me as well.

151

The relationship changes

Expecting a baby for the first time is something entirely new for both him and her. The relationship between the man and the woman of course changes when two become three. There is no way of predicting how pregnancy and parenthood will affect the relationship, just that it will affect it. A good relationship can get better, but it can also become more uncertain. A bad relationship can get even worse, but it can also be strengthened now that it is serious, now that it really counts.

A relationship you thought was a stable one can be shaken hard. It is not unusual that the man feels "cornered." Sometimes he can even leave his pregnant partner for another. It is common to have more fights during pregnancy because it is so important for the relationship to work. We are so afraid that it will not last that even small disagreements scare us. It has to work, now that we will be three. In this way we become more vulnerable to one another.

Living in the present and in the past

A whole lot of old things can come back because of the situation being so new. The relationships to others change particularly when we become pregnant, including the relationship with mom and dad, the siblings, the family of the partner, friends, and colleagues. Now we begin to observe those who have children and those who do not. Even the relationship with pets is altered. Mostly, it is the relationship with one's own parents that changes. As a result of getting pregnant, many tackle the relationship with mom and dad. If it has been good, it might not be necessary to worry so much. However, if the relationship has been bad, thoughts will arise. Why did this happen and what kind of parent will I be? Many find their way back to their parents when they have children. It might perhaps not be such a great relationship, but still tolerable. Sometimes, the grandchild can become a link and mom and dad can become good grandparents. Others are unable to act as grandparents. This may feel very sad.

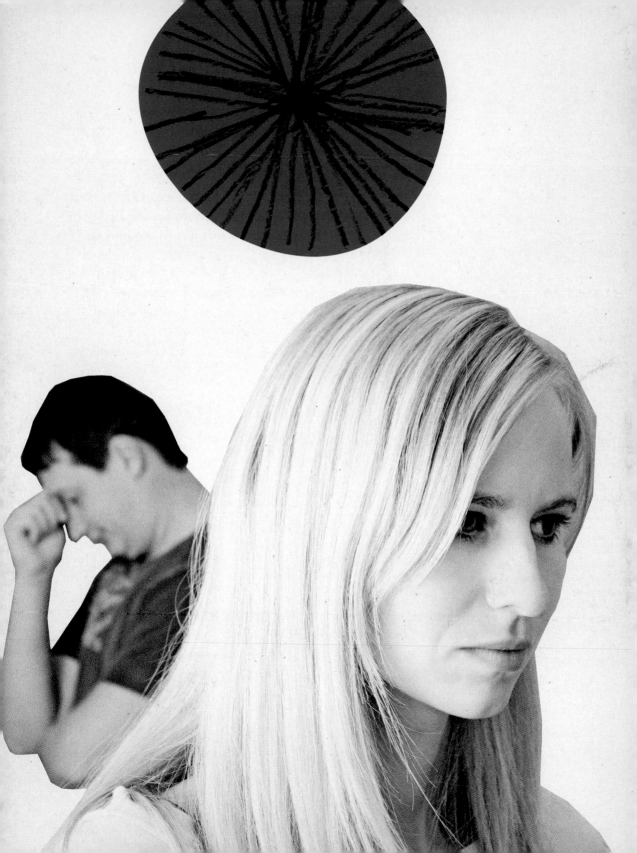

Dealing with things from the past can be frightening. But it is also necessary and is a way to become mature and prepare for parenthood. To reflect upon one's own childhood and the relationship with mom and dad is something that usually happens on its own sooner or later. If it does not happen during pregnancy, it happens later on when the child is born. Perhaps we feel no greater need to "settle accounts" with the past. It is not necessary to work through all of it. One can still be reconciled with the past and move on. If one has had a hard time as a child, it takes extraordinary courage to get pregnant and keep the baby despite one's own experiences.

The self-image changes

As a result of getting pregnant, most women change their way of life. They do not drink, they do not smoke, and they take care of themselves in a different way than before. Some no longer want to fly or drive fast, and some might be more sensitive to watching violent movies. Pregnancy also makes us change the image we have of ourselves. Who am I, what do I want, how am I towards others? And above all, what sort of parent will I become?

Pregnancy is a time when you grow into your new identity as a mother or father. Previously one has been a child, a sister, a friend, and a partner. Now something completely new and very important is expected. Many future parents change their way of life. They think a lot about how their baby will be and look like. One must sort of link together the image of an ordinary baby with the image of the partner to be able to imagine what the baby will be like. It has been shown that when women talk about their expected child they

Maria, thirty-two years old

It was a huge transformation to get pregnant. Previously, my job and my career were my identity. When I became pregnant, at first I felt as if I was skinless. Then I got new skin! It was absolutely amazing!

154

give it more of the traits of its future father than mother. For dads it is the opposite. When dads are asked what sex they want the child to be, it is more common that they want it to be a boy, while moms often imagine a girl.

Some prospective parents excitedly plan for their baby; they buy everything that is needed, and they sew, carve, paint, and arrange a changing table. The drawers are full of tiny clothes. Others do not dare to plan at all. But usually it turns out that they plan some anyway, at least in their mind.

Helena, twenty-seven years old

My mother was an absent mother. She had a career and was not able to give me and my siblings the time and love that we needed. Now I have two children of my own, and she is the most amazing grandmother to them. It feels like reconciliation. I think it is as important to her as it is to me and my children.

Pink clouds and black holes

Some women experience pregnancy as a great time, exactly as they could dream of it. Others experience it as a time of chaos and anxiety, and they feel sick and are almost beaten to the ground by fatigue. Most feel substantially good but they have periods in which they feel worse, physically or psychologically. Even men can get pregnancy symptoms such as nausea and fatigue.

They way the pregnancy turns out is not always linked with how eagerly awaited the baby is. It may rather depend on who you are and what you have been through, and on the relationship to the prospective father or your own parents. Expectations also affect pregnancy. If a friend has had a disabled child or if a sister had a child who died at birth, it increases one's own turmoil. The way you feel in your body also has its affects. Fatigue and nausea can be severe strains.

One thing is for sure: We do not know in advance how we will react and how the pregnancy will be. The same woman can experience different pregnancies in completely different ways. We can be as prepared as we like but it will still not be as we thought it would be.

155

Some women may feel that they lose their own identity when they become pregnant. They are no longer the talented professional women with an abundant social life, but also someone who is about to become a mother. Now the experience in meetings is no longer an advantage. This can lead to a change in one's own self-image and lead to a falter in self-confidence. Obviously, there can also be things than happen during pregnancy that can make the mother feel bad. For example, a loved one who suffers from a disease, or the partner who loses his job or leaves her.

The baby will do well

We often hear that the most important thing for the baby is that the mother feels good during pregnancy, and that worries and anxieties make the baby feel bad. But it has been shown that mothers who are forced to lie in a hospital during the later stages of pregnancy, due to the risk of losing their baby, have children who scream less than other children, even though the mothers of course have been very worried. Nothing suggests that women who, for example, have been left when they were pregnant have more uneasy children than others.

The arguments of the mother and father do not hurt the baby. On the contrary, when the child is born, it knows that this is the way it can be, that this belongs to everyday life.

There is no miracle cure for bad feelings when you are pregnant. On the contrary, we can say that it is good to feel a little bad, to sometimes feel blue and sad. There is sense in reflecting on old and new relationships; this is a way to prepare for being a new and mature person. If one does not ponder during pregnancy, it usually happens when the child is born.

THINGS TO CONSIDER

→ It's good to lose control sometimes and to change. Then you grow as a person and become a better parent.

→ All sorts of thoughts are valuable during pregnancy, both cheerful and happy, sad and worried.

→ It may feel awkward and scary to "come to terms with the past," for example, with one's own parents. But this is a way to becoming mature and to develop, and to become a good parent.

→ It is common to quarrel more during pregnancy, because the relationship changes when two will become three. Now it has to work. You become more vulnerable to one another. The child is not feeling bad about that quarrel.

→ Talking about your thoughts and ruminations with someone you trust or writing them down is good.

→ Accept if you feel small and needy and be open to receive help and care.

→ It is common to feel bad sometimes. It is a way to develop.

→ Seek help if you are struggling. Talk to your midwife or ask to speak with the psychologist at the antenatal clinic.

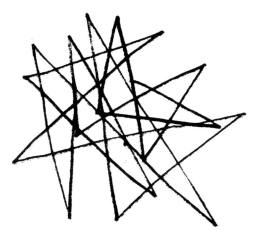

Malin Alfvén is a licensed psychologist and she has worked for many years as a child and parenting psychologist. She frequently lectures for parents and writes the Q&A section of the magazine *We Parents* and has been featured on the Swedish Radio Kiddie Hour. She has written the book *Ask Malin*. Along with Elisabeth Henning and Viveka Holmertz, she has written the *Cesarean Book,* and together with Louise Hallin the book, *Huey Hour.*

Kristina Hofsten is a journalist and has been a writing about children and parents in the *We Parents* magazine for twenty-five years. She has written the *Children's Guide* and *Children In the Beginning.* Together with Lena Lidbeck she has written *The Big Book of Children.*

Index

649.1 ALFVEN

Alfven, Malin.
Time out!

SOF

R4002236356

SOUTH FULTON BRANCH
Atlanta-Fulton Public Library